# GUT INSTINCTS

## A Clinician's Handbook of
## Digestive and Liver Diseases

# GUT INSTINCTS

## A Clinician's Handbook of Digestive and Liver Diseases

Edited by

## Eric Esrailian, MD, MPH
Vice-Chief, Division of Digestive Diseases
Assistant Clinical Professor of Medicine
David Geffen School of Medicine at UCLA
Los Angeles, California

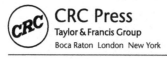

**CRC Press**
Taylor & Francis Group
Boca Raton London New York

CRC Press is an imprint of the
Taylor & Francis Group, an **informa** business

First published 2012 by SLACK Incorporated

Published 2024 by CRC Press
2385 NW Executive Center Drive, Suite 320, Boca Raton FL 33431

and by CRC Press
4 Park Square, Milton Park, Abingdon, Oxon, OX14 4RN

*CRC Press is an imprint of Taylor & Francis Group, LLC*

© 2012 Taylor & Francis Group, LLC

Library of Congress Cataloging-in-Publication Data

Gut instincts : a clinician's handbook of digestive and liver diseases / [edited by] Eric Esrailian.
  p. ; cm.
Includes bibliographical references and index.
ISBN 978-1-55642-977-4 (alk. paper)
1. Gastrointestinal system--Diseases--Handbooks, manuals, etc. 2. Liver--Diseases--Handbooks, manuals, etc. I. Esrailian, Eric.
[DNLM: 1. Gastrointestinal Diseases--diagnosis--Handbooks. 2. Gastrointestinal Diseases--therapy--Handbooks. 3. Liver Diseases--diagnosis--Handbooks. 4. Liver Diseases--therapy--Handbooks. WI 39]
RC801.G88 2012
616.3'62--dc23
                                2011025319

ISBN: 9781556429774 (pbk)
ISBN: 9781003524489 (ebk)

DOI: 10.1201/9781003524489

# Dedication

To Melina, Derek, and Andrew. You inspire and strengthen me beyond words. I am truly blessed.

# Contents

# Acknowledgments

This text has been a labor of love, and I am grateful to my amazing group of co-authors for dedicating their time and talents to this valuable educational project. My deepest thanks go out to my wife and children who enthusiastically put up with my late nights, early mornings, and everything in-between. My parents deserve special thanks for their unconditional support over the years and for the sacrifices they have made for their children. I am grateful to the patients who have allowed me to learn from them and who continue to teach me every day; it is an honor to be able to care for them. I am also grateful to the countless colleagues, fellows, residents, and students I have been fortunate to work with over the years. Important thanks to 2 unique high school teachers, Sue Black and Milo Gwosden, who exemplify what it means to teach, and I carry around lessons I learned from them even to this day. I would like to thank Bruce Runyon for being my first mentor, for seeing something in me as a medical student, and for stimulating my interest in academic medicine. Special thanks goes to Carrie Kotlar for her dedication to making this book a reality. I also owe thanks to friends and colleagues Bennett Roth, Fred Weinstein, Brennan Spiegel, and Simon Beaven for being the best at what they do, and being even better friends along the way. I would like to specifically thank my mentor and dear friend, Gary Gitnick, for his support, guidance, and for continually pushing me to reach for the next level. Finally, I would like to thank Kirk Kerkorian—on behalf of all Armenians throughout the world—for his unsurpassed support of humanity.

# About the Editor

*Eric Esrailian, MD, MPH* is the Vice-Chief of the Division of Digestive Diseases and an Assistant Clinical Professor of Medicine at the David Geffen School of Medicine at the University of California-Los Angeles (UCLA). The UCLA Division of Digestive Diseases is among the largest and most historic of such divisions in the world.

Attending the University of California at Berkeley and graduating with a major in Integrative Biology and a minor in English, he subsequently graduated from the Loma Linda University School of Medicine and completed a residency in internal medicine at the University of Southern California.

Dr. Esrailian was named intern, junior resident, and senior resident of the year during all 3 years of his residency training. He completed his gastroenterology fellowship at UCLA where he also obtained a Masters of Public Health degree with the assistance of a NIH-sponsored training grant. He is also a graduate of the Executive Program in Management from the UCLA Anderson School of Management. He has authored or co-authored manuscripts, book chapters, and abstracts on various topics within digestive and liver diseases, and his primary clinical interests include gastrointestinal endoscopy, inflammatory bowel diseases, gastrointestinal hemorrhage, and functional gastrointestinal diseases such as irritable bowel syndrome.

In 2010, Dr. Esrailian was appointed to the Medical Board of California by Governor Arnold Schwarzenegger.

# Contributing Authors

*Gillian M. Barlow, PhD (Chapter 22)*
Research Associate III
Division of Gastroenterology
Department of Medicine
Cedars-Sinai Medical Center
Los Angeles, California

*Simon W. Beaven, MD, PhD (Chapter 32)*
Assistant Professor
Division of Digestive Diseases
Pfleger Liver Institute
David Geffen School of Medicine at UCLA
Los Angeles, California

*Yasser M. Bhat, MD (Chapter 13)*
Medical Director, Esophageal Imaging and Therapy
California Pacific Medical Center
Director, Interventional Endoscopy
San Francisco VA Medical Center
Assistant Clinical Professor of Medicine
University of California San Francisco
San Francisco, California

*Lin Chang, MD (Chapter 20)*
Professor of Medicine
Co-Director, Center for Neurobiology of Stress
David Geffen School of Medicine at UCLA
Los Angeles, California

*William D. Chey, MD, AGAF, FACG, FACP (Chapter 11)*
Director, GI Physiology Laboratory
Co-Director, Michigan Bowel Control Program
University of Michigan Health System
Ann Arbor, Michigan

*Daniel D. Cho, MD (Chapter 2)*
Assistant Clinical Professor
Department of Medicine
Division of Digestive Diseases
David Geffen School of Medicine at UCLA
Los Angeles, California

*Jeffrey L. Conklin, MD, FACG (Chapter 4)*
Director, Esophageal Center
Professor of Medicine
Division of Gastroenterology and Hepatology
Cedars-Sinai Medical Center
Los Angeles, California

*Lynn Shapiro Connolly, MD (Chapter 19)*
Gastroenterology Fellow
Division of Digestive Diseases
David Geffen School of Medicine at UCLA
Los Angeles, California

*Stanley Dea, MD (Chapter 8)*
Chief of Gastroenterology
Olive View-UCLA Medical Center
Clinical Professor of Medicine
David Geffen School of Medicine at UCLA
Los Angeles, California

*John A. Donovan, MD (Chapter 36)*
Assistant Professor of Clinical Medicine
Division of Gastrointestinal and Liver Diseases
Department of Medicine
Keck School of Medicine
University of Southern California
Los Angeles, California

*Marla Dubinsky, MD (Chapter 17)*
Associate Professor of Pediatrics
Director of the Pediatric IBD Center
Cedars-Sinai Medical Center
Los Angeles, California

*John P. Duffy, MD (Chapter 42)*
Hepatobiliary and Abdominal Transplant Surgeon
Nazih Zuhdi Transplant Institute
Integris Baptist Medical Center
Oklahoma City, Oklahoma

*Francisco Antonio Durazo, MD, FACP (Chapter 38)*
Associate Professor of Medicine and Surgery
Medical Director, UCLA Liver Transplant Program
David Geffen School of Medicine at UCLA
Los Angeles, California

*Erik P. Dutson, MD, FACS (Chapter 15)*
Associate Professor of Surgery
David Geffen School of Medicine at UCLA
Department of Surgery
UCLA Ronald Reagan Medical Center
Los Angeles, California

*James Farrell, MD (Chapter 12)*
Director of Endoscopic Ultrasound
Associate Professor of Medicine
Division of Digestive Diseases
David Geffen School of Medicine at UCLA
Los Angeles, California

*Kevin A. Ghassemi, MD (Chapters 9 and 44)*
Clinical Instructor of Gastroenterology
Division of Digestive Diseases
David Geffen School of Medicine at UCLA
Los Angeles, California

*Terri Getzug, MD (Chapter 1)*
Associate Clinical Professor of Medicine
Division of Digestive Diseases
David Geffen School of Medicine at UCLA
Los Angeles, California

*Steven-Huy Han, MD, AGAF (Chapter 33)*
Professor of Medicine and Surgery
Pfleger Liver Institute
David Geffen School of Medicine at UCLA
Los Angeles, California

*O. Joe Hines, MD (Chapter 28)*
Professor of Surgery
Department of Surgery
David Geffen School of Medicine at UCLA
Los Angeles, California

*Wendy Ho, MD, MPH (Chapter 45)*
Assistant Clinical Professor of Medicine
Division of Digestive Diseases
David Geffen School of Medicine at UCLA
Los Angeles, California

*Ke-Qin Hu, MD (Chapter 34)*
Director, Hepatology Services
Professor of Clinical Medicine
Division of Gastroenterology/Hepatology
University of California
Irvine Medical Center
Orange, California

*Dennis M. Jensen, MD (Chapter 9)*
Professor of Medicine
David Geffen School of Medicine at UCLA
Division of Digestive Diseases
UCLA Medical Centet
West Los Angeles VA Medical Center
CURE Digestive Diseases Research Center
Los Angeles, California

*Rome Jutabha, MD (Chapter 23)*
Professor of Medicine
Division of Digestive Diseases
David Geffen School of Medicine at UCLA
Ronald Reagan UCLA Medical Center
Los Angeles, California

*Fasiha Kanwal, MS, MSHS (Chapter 37)*
Associate Professor of Medicine
John Cochran VA Medical Center
School of Medicine, St. Louis University
Department of Gastroenterology and Hepatology
St. Louis, Missouri

*Theodoros Kelesidis, MD (Chapter 26)*
Department of Medicine, Division of Infectious Diseases
Ronald Reagan Medical Center
University of California Los Angeles
Los Angeles, California

*Saro Khemichian, MD (Chapter 36)*
Clinical Instructor
Division of Gastrointestinal and Liver Diseases
Department of Medicine
Keck School of Medicine
University of Southern California
Los Angeles, California

*Vandana Khungar, MD, MSc (Chapters 33 and 41)*
Gastroenterology Fellow
Cedars-Sinai Medical Center
Department of Gastroenterology and Hepatology
Los Angeles, California

*Kunut Kijsirichareanchai, MD (Chapter 23)*
Resident Instructor
Department of Internal Medicine
Texas Tech University Health Science Center
Lubbock, Texas

*Thomas O. G. Kovacs, MD (Chapter 10)*
Professor of Medicine
David Geffen School of Medicine at UCLA
Division of Digestive Diseases
VA Greater Los Angeles Health Care System
Los Angeles, California

*Amy Lightner, MD (Chapter 31)*
Resident in General Surgery
David Geffen School of Medicine at UCLA
Department of Surgery
Ronald Reagan UCLA Medical Center
Los Angeles, California

*Emeran A. Mayer, MD (Chapter 21)*
Professor of Medicine, Physiology and Psychiatry
David Geffen School of Medicine at UCLA
Division of Digestive Diseases
Los Angeles, California

*Gil Y. Melmed, MD, MS (Chapter 16)*
Assistant Clinical Professor of Medicine
David Geffen School of Medicine at UCLA
Division of Gastroenterology
Cedars-Sinai Medical Center
Los Angeles, California

*Michel H. Mendler, MD, MS (Chapter 35)*
Associate Professor of Medicine
Loma Linda University Medical Center
Division of Gastroenterology and Hepatology
Transplantation Institute and Liver Center
Loma Linda, California

*Lilah F. Morris, MD (Chapter 28)*
Resident in Surgery
Department of Surgery
David Geffen School of Medicine at UCLA
Los Angeles, California

*Udayakumar Navaneethan, MD (Chapter 18)*
Gastroenterology Fellow
Digestive Disease Institute
The Cleveland Clinic
Cleveland, Ohio

*Vivian Ng, MD (Chapter 39)*
Department of Medicine
David Geffen School of Medicine at UCLA
Los Angeles, California

*Mark Ovsiowitz, MD (Chapter 3)*
Assistant Clinical Professor of Medicine
Division of Digestive Diseases
Department of Medicine
David Geffen School of Medicine at UCLA
Los Angeles, California

*David A. Pegues, MD (Chapter 27)*
Professor of Clinical Medicine
David Geffen School of Medicine at UCLA
Division of Infectious Diseases
Ronald Reagan UCLA Medical Center
Los Angeles, California

*Mark Pimentel, MD, FRCP(C) (Chapter 22)*
Director, GI Motility Program
Associate Professor of Medicine
Cedars-Sinai Medical Center
Los Angeles, California

*Charalabos Pothoulakis, MD (Chapter 26)*
Eli and Edythe Broad Professor of Medicine
Department of Medicine, Division of Digestive Diseases
Ronald Reagan Medical Center
Los Angeles, California

*Bennett E. Roth, MD (Chapter 5)*
Professor of Clinical Medicine
Chief, Clinical Affairs
Division of Digestive Diseases
David Geffen School of Medicine at UCLA
Los Angeles, California

*Bruce A. Runyon, MD (Chapter 40)*
Professor of Medicine
Loma Linda University Medical Center
Loma Linda, California

*Sammy Saab, MD, MPH, AGAF (Chapter 39)*
Associate Professor of Medicine
Surgery Assistant Professor of Nursing Head
Outcomes Research in Hepatology
David Geffen School of Medicine at UCLA
Los Angeles, California

*Richard J. Saad, MD, MS (Chapter 11)*
Assistant Professor of Medicine
Division of Gastroenterology
University of Michigan Hospital and Health Systems
Ann Arbor, Michigan

*Jonathan Sack, MD (Chapters 29 and 30)*
Associate Clinical Professor of Surgery
David Geffen School of Medicine at UCLA
Department of Surgery
Ronald Reagan UCLA Medical Center
Los Angeles, California

*Saeed Sadeghi, MD (Chapter 24)*
Assistant Clinical Professor of Medicine
Division of Hematology and Oncology
David Geffen School of Medicine at UCLA
Los Angeles, California

*Bo Shen, MD, FACG (Chapter 18)*
Professor of Medicine
Digestive Disease Institute
Department of Gastroenterology and Hepatology
The Cleveland Clinic
Cleveland, Ohio

*Inder M. Singh, MD (Chapter 13)*
Clinical Fellow
David Geffen School of Medicine at UCLA
University of California Los Angeles
Division of Digestive Diseases
Los Angeles, California

*Tram T. Tran, MD (Chapter 41)*
Medical Director, Liver Transplantation
Cedars-Sinai Medical Center
Los Angeles, California

*Leo Treyzon, MD, MS (Chapter 7)*
Clinical Instructor
David Geffen School of Medicine at UCLA
Division of Digestive Diseases
Cedars Sinai Medical Center
Los Angeles, California

*Zev A. Wainberg, MD, MSc (Chapter 6)*
Assisant Professor of Medicine
Division of Hematology/Oncology
David Geffen School of Medicine at UCLA
Los Angeles, California

*Samuel H. Wald, MD (Chapter 43)*
Clinical Professor of Anesthesiology
David Geffen School of Medicine at UCLA
Los Angeles, California

*Wilfred M. Weinstein, MD (Chapter 14)*
Professor of Medicine
Division of Digestive Diseases
David Geffen School of Medicine at UCLA
Los Angeles, California

*Jeremy M. Wong, MD (Chapter 43)*
Assistant Clinical Professor of Anesthesiology
David Geffen School of Medicine at UCLA
Los Angeles, California

*James Yoo, MD, FACS, FASCRS (Chapter 31)*
Assistant Professor
Chief, Section of Colon & Rectal Surgery
David Geffen School of Medicine at UCLA
Department of Surgery
Ronald Reagan UCLA Medical Center
Los Angeles, California

*David Da Zheng, BS (Chapter 15)*
Medical Student
Medical College of Wisconsin
Milwaukee, Wisconsin

# Preface

*Gut Instincts* was carefully designed to meet an important need for practicing clinicians, health care providers, and trainees—a convenient handbook that answers the "what should I know?" and "what should I do?" questions that we all face while treating patients. An impressive collection of expert clinicians and academic-thought leaders have come together to impart their knowledge of evidence-based medicine and clinical pearls in a concise format that can be accessed in the office or at the bedside.

*Gut Instincts* covers the most frequently encountered digestive and liver disease problems seen in clinical practice. The focus of each chapter is diagnosis and management, and a few key references are provided for further study and review. I often explain to patients how we all have "gut instincts" and "gut feelings." Each chapter of this book contains a "gut instincts" section with 5 key pearls for the reader to remember. We often teach students with "take-home points," and the gut instincts sections summarize these points. Every chapter also has an important table, figure, or algorithm that will help readers learn and remember important concepts for patient care.

As modern providers, we have an unprecedented amount of information at our fingertips and diminishing amounts of time to spend with patients. *Gut Instincts* aims to help us make the best decisions for our patients in a practical and efficient manner. Although it is not intended to replace a comprehensive textbook on the bookshelf, *Gut Instincts* will be a valued complement for anyone who treats or studies digestive and liver diseases.

# Foreword

The study of digestive diseases in the 21st century emanates from an explosion of knowledge as a result of dramatic advances in the basic sciences coupled with an enormous array of translational studies yielding clinical guidelines based on outcomes assessment. The modern management of digestive diseases, in large part, is now based on the results of well-designed prospective controlled trials. Nevertheless, in practice, the accumulated wisdom of experts with judgment, which comes from experience, remains essential to the art of the practice of clinical gastroenterology. This book is a practical compendium of modern accumulated knowledge, coupled with wisdom and judgment based on the experience of experts. The dramatic growth and accumulated knowledge has resulted in extensive modifications of established practices requiring that practitioners of the management of digestive diseases regularly revise and review their management of patients in light of new information and new insights. *Gut Instincts* has been prepared by leaders in the practical application of modern concepts of the management of digestive diseases. The volume of new information challenges contributors to be succinct while still providing a practical approach to modern clinical management. This book organizes and incorporates biomedical information in digestive diseases and presents it in a compact, thoroughly practical, and readable format. It is a relatively short, but authoritative, source for consultation for the busy clinician, and it provides the essential basis upon which a true consultation in gastroenterology can emanate. *Gut Instincts* bridges the gap between large encyclopedic textbooks and multiple reviews of diverse areas of digestive diseases, and it is practical, user-friendly, and convenient for the busy clinician. Although the emphasis is on therapy rather than on theory, the book appropriately provides guidelines based on established pathophysiology, clinical and laboratory diagnosis, and differential diagnosis. This practical handbook is enriched with the contributions of younger authors, as well as established clinicians, all being experts in their special fields. Readers will hopefully be able to avoid unnecessary and costly tests but still provide patients with the benefits of modern diagnosis. The practice of clinical gastroenterology is an art as well as a science. Much remains based on instinct and experience as well as modern outcomes assessment. *Gut Instincts* combines elements of all of the above to guide the clinician to provide the highest level of excellence in delivery of care to patients with digestive diseases.

*Gary Gitnick, MD, FACG*
Chief, Division of Digestive Diseases
Professor of Medicine
David Geffen School of Medicine at UCLA
Los Angeles, California

# UPPER GASTROINTESTINAL TRACT

# CHAPTER 1

# NAUSEA AND VOMITING

TERRI GETZUG, MD

Nausea and vomiting are common and distressing symptoms with a number of underlying causes. Nausea may or may not be accompanied by vomiting or other symptoms. Vomiting is the forceful expulsion of gastric contents through the mouth. Vomiting may also occur in the absence of nausea in some settings. Regurgitation is passive and relates to the return of esophageal contents into the mouth. The differential diagnosis is extensive and includes a broad range of conditions from within and outside the gut, as well as from drugs and circulating toxins.

## Pathophysiology

Vomiting is coordinated by the brainstem and is effected by neuromuscular responses in the gut. The cerebral cortex is involved, and nausea requires conscious perception. Several brainstem nuclei coordinate the initiation of vomiting. Emetic stimuli can act at several sites, such as the cerebral cortex (provoked by unpleasant thoughts or smells), the labyrinthine apparatus (motion sickness/inner ear disorders), vagal afferent nerves (gastric irritants), and nongastric visceral afferents (intestinal and colonic obstruction/mesenteric ischemia). The medulla contains the chemoreceptor trigger zone, which senses bloodborne emetic stimuli and metabolic factors.

Esrailian E. *Gut Instincts: A Clinician's Handbook of Digestive and Liver Diseases* (pp 3-10).
© 2012 Taylor & Francis Group

# Clinical Approach to Nausea and Vomiting

## HISTORY

The patient history is critical, and most patients have symptoms, signs, or basic laboratory results that point to the etiology. Symptom duration is critical to the differential diagnosis of acute versus chronic nausea and vomiting. Acute onset suggests an acute process such as a toxin, infection, pancreatitis, cholecystitis, or a drug-related side effect. Symptoms lasting longer than 1 month are considered chronic. Timing (morning, postprandial either immediate or delayed, with or without nausea) and description of the emesis (undigested or partially digested, bilious, bloody, feculent) should be noted. Relief of abdominal pain by vomiting characterizes a small bowel obstruction (SBO), but has no effect on pain from inflammatory processes such as pancreatitis or cholecystitis. The clinician should also ask about associated symptoms such as vertigo, diarrhea, fever, weight loss, headache, and early satiety.

## PHYSICAL EXAMINATION

Orthostasis and tachycardia are associated with volume depletion. A general physical examination can detect signs such as jaundice, lymphadenopathy, abdominal masses, occult blood in the stool, and features of thyrotoxicosis or adrenal insufficiency. The abdominal examination is critical. Attention should be paid to the degree of distention; hernias; visible peristalsis; presence of a succussion splash; quality of bowel sounds (high-pitched, tinkling, or absent); and the presence of tenderness, guarding, or rebound. Loss of dental enamel or calluses on the dorsum of the hands might point to bulimia. Fundoscopic examination may reveal papilledema. Neurologic examination may show nystagmus or evidence of neuropathy. A third heart sound or bilateral pulmonary crackles may indicate heart failure. The patient's affect may suggest depression or anxiety.

## Causes

Adverse reactions to medications are among the most common causes. Usually, nausea from a drug presents early in the treatment course. Many classes can induce nausea. Drugs evoke vomiting by action on the stomach (analgesics, erythromycin) or medulla (digoxin, opiates, anti-Parkinsonian drugs). Other emetogenic drugs include antibiotics, cardiac anti-arrhythmics, oral hypoglycemics, and contraceptives. Chemotherapy can cause acute vomiting (within hours of use), delayed (after 1 or more days), or anticipatory. Acute vomiting is mediated by 5-HT3 (serotonin) pathways, whereas delayed emesis is 5-HT3 independent. Anticipatory nausea often responds best to anxiolytics. Marijuana has been associated with recurrent vomiting with features similar to cyclic vomiting syndrome.

Infections are also common etiologies. Acute gastroenteritis can be caused by bacteria, viruses, and parasites and is often characterized by diarrhea, vomiting, or both. Vomiting is common with rotaviruses, enteric adenovirus, and Norwalk agent. Bacterial infections with *Staphylococcus aureus*, *Salmonella*, *Bacillus cereus*, and *Clostridium perfringens* also produce symptoms via toxins acting on the brainstem. Otitis media, meningitis, and hepatitis are a few common nongastrointestinal infections associated with nausea.

Nausea, vomiting, and vertigo are common symptoms associated with labyrinthine disorders. Motion sickness, viral labyrinthitis, Meniere's disease, and tumors can all cause vomiting. Nausea and vomiting may complicate 10% to 70% of surgical procedures. Risk factors include female gender, younger age, nonsmoker status, and opioids.

Obstructions produce nausea, which may be relieved by vomiting. Symptoms from a gastric outlet obstruction may be intermittent, whereas a SBO is generally acute and associated with abdominal pain, distention, and tenderness. Bowel obstructions occur from adhesions, tumors, volvulus, intussusception, fecal impaction, or inflammatory bowel disease. Gastroparesis and pseudo-obstruction are functional disorders, that can mimic obstruction without an anatomic lesion. Gastroparesis may be related to a systemic disease (diabetes, scleroderma, lupus, amyloidosis, postgastric surgery) or may be idiopathic (viral, postinfectious paraneoplastic, functional dyspepsia, psychiatric disorders). Intestinal pseudo-obstruction may be idiopathic, inherited (familial visceral myopathy or neuropathy), from systemic disease (scleroderma), or part of a paraneoplastic syndrome. Other functional disorders include chronic idiopathic nausea, functional vomiting, and cyclic vomiting syndrome, which is often associated with migraine headaches.

Pancreatitis, appendicitis, cholecystitis, and biliary colic may cause symptoms by activation of visceral afferent nerves that promote ileus. Fulminant liver failure may cause symptoms via an emetic toxin and elevated intracranial pressure. Any disorder increasing intracranial pressure may produce emesis even without nausea. Migraines, seizures, emotional responses (to unpleasant smells, tastes, or memories), and psychiatric disorders (anxiety, eating disorders, depression) may promote symptoms.

Metabolic disorders including uremia, ketoacidosis, adrenal insufficiency, and parathyroid/thyroid disease can cause nausea and vomiting as can pregnancy (70% to 85% of pregnant women in the first trimester). It is important to remember that myocardial infarction and congestive heart failure can also present with digestive symptoms.

## Diagnostic Evaluation

The diagnostic evaluation should be guided by the duration, frequency, and severity of symptoms. Blood tests for electrolytes, glucose, renal function, and complete blood count should initially be obtained if symptoms persist. If abdominal pain is present, additional studies should include pancreatic enzymes, liver tests, pregnancy testing, and drug levels.

Abdominal plain films may show obstruction or ileus but may be unrevealing in many patients with documented SBO. Anatomic studies may be indicated if initial tests are nondiagnostic. Upper endoscopy may reveal tumors, ulcers, and mucosal disorders. Small bowel follow-through or computed tomography enterography may demonstrate reasons for a partial or complete bowel obstruction; inflammatory disorders; masses; or pancreatic, hepatobiliary, or retroperitoneal pathology. Abdominal ultrasound can show gallstones. Colonic contrast enemas or colonoscopy may reveal a source for colonic obstruction. Magnetic resonance imaging/magnetic resonance angiography may suggest mesenteric ischemia or superior mesenteric compression syndrome. A radionuclide gastric emptying study is the most commonly used screening test of gastric motor function. However, abnormal gastric emptying does not necessarily prove cause-and-effect with symptoms. Antroduodenal manometry and electrogastrography are available only in referral centers, and the utility of these modalities is unclear.

## Treatment

There are 3 basic principles to remember: (1) correct any fluid, electrolyte, or nutritional deficiencies; (2) identify and eliminate the underlying cause; and (3) suppress or eliminate the symptoms even if the primary cause cannot be identified. A nasogastric tube may need to be placed for decompression with gastric distention or bowel obstruction. Dietary manipulation may be helpful. Fat and fiber should be avoided in the setting of gastroparesis because they delay gastric emptying.

Antiemetics and prokinetics are 2 broad therapeutic categories (Table 1-1). Antiemetics affect the central nervous system. These include phenothiazine dopamine antagonists (prochlorperazine), tricyclic antidepressants (nortryptaline), and serotonin 5-HT3 antagonists

| TABLE 1-1 | TREATMENT OF NAUSEA AND VOMITING | | |
|---|---|---|---|
| **Drug Class** | **Mechanism** | **Examples** | **Uses** |
| Antiemetic | Dopamine antagonist | Proclorperazine, Chlorpromazine | Multiple indications including gastroenteritis, medications, toxins, postoperative, radiation |
| | Anticholinergic | Scopalamine | Motion sickness, inner ear disease |
| | Antihistamine | Meclizine, Diphenhydramine | Motion sickness, inner ear disease |
| | Tricyclic antidepressant | Amitriptyline, nortriptyline | Chronic idiopathic nausea, functional vomiting, cyclic vomiting syndrome, diabetic gastropathy |
| | 5-HT3 antagonist | Ondansetron | Chemotherapy- and radiation-induced emesis, postoperative, AIDS |
| Antiemetic/ prokinetic | 5-HT4 agonist, dopamine antagonist | Metoclopramide | Gastroparesis |
| | Peripheral dopamine antagonist | Domperidone | Gastroparesis |
| Prokinetic | Motilin agonist | Erythromycin | Gastroparesis, intestinal pseudo-obstruction |
| | 5-HT4 agonist | Tegaserod | Gastroparesis, pseudo-obstruction |
| | Muscarinic agonist | Bethanechol | Gastroparesis |
| | Somatostatin analogue | Octreotide | Intestinal pseudo-obstruction |

*(continued)*

| TABLE 1-1 | TREATMENT OF NAUSEA AND VOMITING (CONTINUED) | | |
|-----------|----------------------------------------------|---|---|
| **Drug Class** | **Mechanism** | **Examples** | **Uses** |
| Special alternatives | Glucocorticoid | Dexamethasone, methylprednisolone | Chemotherapy-induced emesis |
| | Benzodiazepine | Lorazepam | Anticipatory nausea and vomiting with chemotherapy |
| | Cannabinoid | Tetrahydro-cannabinol | Chemotherapy-induced emesis, AIDS |
| | Botulinum toxin | | Pyloric stenosis, gastroparesis |
| | Ginger, accupressure, hypnosis | | Nausea and vomiting |
| | Psychotherapy | | Bulimia, rumination syndrome, psychogenic causes of nausea and vomiting |

(ondansetron). Corticosteroids (dexamethasone) have also been used in combination with other agents to treat chemotherapy-related symptoms. Prokinetics peripherally alter gastric motor function or reflex activity. Examples include metoclopramide, domperidone, bethanechol, and erythromycin. Effectiveness of newer 5-HT4 agonists is being evaluated. Antihistamines, cannabinoids, octreotide, and benzodiazepines are also useful in specific clinical scenarios. Selected gastroparesis patients may benefit from pyloric botulinum toxin injection and surgically-placed gastric neurostimulators. Complementary treatments using ginger, acupressure, hypnosis, and psychotherapy have also shown some efficacy in clinical trials.

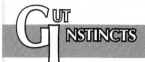

## Nausea and Vomiting

1. The complications of nausea and vomiting (fluid depletion, hypokalemia, metabolic alkalosis) should be recognized and treated immediately.
2. A careful history and physical examination can often uncover the cause of symptoms.
3. Laboratory evaluation and further diagnostic testing should be guided by symptom duration, frequency, severity, and character of the vomiting episodes and associated symptoms.
4. Targeted therapy to correct underlying medical and surgical problems should be provided and symptoms should be treated.
5. If a patient developed side effects with metoclopramide, domperidone would offer similar clinical benefits with a greatly reduced likelihood of side effects.

## Key References

1. Hasler WL, Chey WD. Nausea and vomiting. *Gastroenterology*. 2003;125(6): 1860-1867.
2. Quigley EM, Hasler WL, Parkman HP. AGA technical review on nausea and vomiting. *Gastroenterology*. 2001;120(1):263-286.

# CHAPTER 2

# Gastroesophageal Reflux Disease

Daniel D. Cho, MD

Gastroesophageal reflux disease (GERD) is one of the most common upper digestive disorders encountered by primary-care physicians and gastroenterologists. The distinction between physiologic and pathologic reflux remains debated. Not surprisingly, the definition and criteria for GERD differs in the literature. The most widely accepted definition is the Montreal definition, which classifies GERD as "a condition which develops when the reflux of gastric contents causes troublesome symptoms and/or complications." What is troublesome is largely up to the perception of the patient, assuming symptoms have caused a notable decrease in quality of life. The presence of erosive esophagitis on esophagogastroduodenoscopy (EGD) is not a prerequisite for the diagnosis of GERD.

## Evaluation

The diagnosis of GERD is largely symptom based with the classical features of heartburn (pyrosis) and regurgitation. Associated symptoms of dysphagia, globus sensation, dysgeusia, and water brash may also be present. GERD can be one of a number of contributing factors to the extraesophageal manifestations of laryngitis, cough, throat clearing, and asthma exacerbation. Often in clinical practice, response to an empirical trial of antacids, histamine-2 blockers, or proton pump inhibitors (PPIs) essentially confirms the diagnosis. Endoscopic evaluation should be

Esrailian E. *Gut Instincts: A Clinician's Handbook of Digestive and Liver Diseases* (pp 11-16). © 2012 Taylor & Francis Group

reserved for patients with symptoms of GERD with dysphagia, those who have failed maximal PPI therapy (bid dosing), and those exhibiting any "red flag" signs or symptoms concerning for occult gastrointestinal malignancy. The issue of screening and surveillance of Barrett's esophagus will be discussed in Chapter 5. Alternative diagnoses should always be considered, which include, but are not limited to, a cardiac etiology, non-GERD–related esophagitis (eosinophilic, infectious, pill-induced), or esophageal motility disorders (achalasia, diffuse esophageal spasm, hypertensive lower esophageal sphincter). Manometry and ambulatory pH/pH-impedance studies are usually reserved for patients with refractory GERD who have had an unremarkable EGD. Current recommendations are for pH studies to be performed while patient stops taking PPIs (for at least 1 week).

## Management

Lifestyle modifications such as weight loss, head of the bed elevation, and avoidance of meals 1 hour prior to bedtime may be beneficial in the appropriate clinical context. Likewise, avoidance of trigger foods such as coffee, alcohol, fatty foods, chocolate, and peppermint may be considered but often can be unrealistic. Smoking cessation should also be advocated.

Studies have shown a clear superiority of PPIs for treatment and maintenance of erosive esophagitis. However, often in clinical practice, practitioners are presented with patients with symptoms of GERD who do not have esophagitis. Antacids are ideal for immediate relief of occasional symptoms. Patients who require short courses of acid suppression often obtain relief with histamine-2 blockers. However, tachyphylaxis with histamine-2 blockers (within weeks to months) limits their consistent use in patients who require long-term acid suppression or as an adjunct to PPI therapy in patients with breakthrough symptoms. It is certainly reasonable to adopt a "step up" approach based on the severity of symptoms. In patients who continue to be symptomatic despite daily dosing of PPIs, bid dosing is recommended. Changing the PPI can also be considered although this is largely based on anecdotal experience. Often, practitioners begin with PPI therapy in which case a "step down" approach should be considered after 1 to 2 months. A recurrence of symptoms within 3 months is seen as an indication for maintenance therapy.

Various prokinetic agents have been utilized in the past to promote gastric acid clearance. The potential for adverse effects has largely limited their use. Use of metoclopramide has been discouraged in light of recent medical-legal uses with movements disorders, such as tardive dyskinesia, with long-term use. Cisapride is no longer available given its risk of cardiac dysrhythmias. Use of bethanechol has never gained wide acceptance given its anticholinergic effects.

Despite the perception that prolonged esophageal acid exposure leads to peptic strictures, Barrett's esophagus, or adenocarcinoma, treatment on an as-needed basis or for short courses based on symptomatology is certainly appropriate. Patients who merely have the symptomatology of GERD very rarely "progress" to metaplasia, dysplasia, or adenocarcinoma of the distal esophagus.

Should patients be refractory to PPI therapy, it is important to remember a few salient points. A PPI is best given 30 minutes prior to meals: (1) for once-daily dosing, prior to breakfast or dinner depending on the timing of symptoms for an individual patient, and (2) for twice-daily dosing, prior to breakfast and dinner. Dexlansoprazole can be taken without regard to food. PPIs are not generally as effective when given at bedtime. You can consider additional testing as mentioned previously. Consider the possibility of esophageal hypersensitivity (which is associated with reflux of nonacidic contents) or functional heartburn (which is not correlated with reflux). Alternative or adjunct therapy includes low-dose tricyclic antidepressants, selective serotonin reuptake inhibitors, or trazadone. There is limited literature supporting baclofen use for transient lower-esophageal sphincter relaxation. These therapies may be limited by adverse effects, particularly depression of the central nervous system. I favor using desipramine starting at 10 mg, which is titrated up by 10 mg every 1 to 2 weeks and given in the evenings to minimize adverse effects. Figure 2-1 outlines the algorithm for the evaluation and treatment of GERD.

## Surgery

Antireflux surgery, specifically laparoscopic Nissen fundoplication, is an attractive therapeutic approach to many patients who require maintenance therapy. Limited studies have shown an advantage of fundoplication to medical therapy for symptoms of heartburn and regurgitation. However, approximately 30% of patients who have reflux surgery are back on medical therapy within 5 years. Although the morbidity with fundoplication is low, a significant number of patients do experience dysphagia requiring endoscopic dilation. Other potential complications include an inability to belch (with flatulence) and a change in bowel habits. This issue is further complicated by the fact that patients who are most likely to have the greatest benefit from fundoplication are those who are well controlled on medical therapy. Current guidelines favor PPIs for maintenance therapy given these

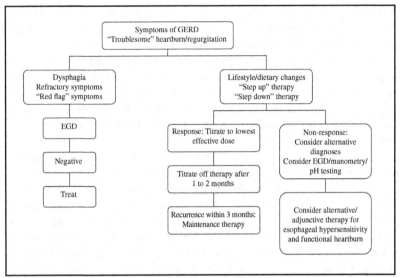

**Figure 2-1.** GERD evaluation and treatment algorithm.

factors. Exceptions include patients who are well controlled on PPIs but have significant adverse medication effects or those patients with a predominance of regurgitation with reflux. Other potential candidates include younger, healthy patients who are well controlled on medical therapy but wish to have surgery to obviate the need for long-term medication use. In patients seeking reflux surgery for GERD-like symptoms refractory to maximal PPI therapy, alternative etiologies should be considered.

## Controversies

The ongoing issue of concomitant PPI and clopidogrel use and increased risk for coronary events remains an important topic. A number of recent conflicting retrospective studies have ensured that this controversy will continue and warrants further research. There does seem to be a small, but measurable increased risk of *Clostridium difficile* colitis, other enteric infections, decreased bone density, and pneumonia with chronic PPI use. Current American Gastroenterological Association guidelines recommend against routine calcium supplementation and dual energy x-ray absorptiometry (DEXA) scans given insufficient evidence. Nonetheless, the lowest effective dose is advocated in the guidelines for chronic acid suppression.

# Pregnancy

New onset and exacerbation of pre-existing GERD is certainly common in pregnancy, particularly through the latter trimesters. Omeprazole is a Class C medication while other PPIs are considered to be in the Class B category. PPIs have not been shown to be associated with teratogenicity or pregnancy complications. Nonetheless, given the longer safety record with histamine-2 blockers, most obstetricians favor this class of medication.

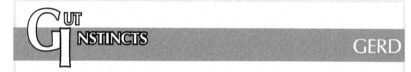

GERD

1. The diagnosis of GERD in clinical practice is largely symptom based. The classical symptoms are heartburn (pyrosis) and regurgitation.

2. Response to empirical trials of antacids, histamine-2 blockers, or PPIs are generally sufficient to confirm the diagnosis.

3. Endoscopic evaluation should be considered in patients with associated dysphagia, in those refractory to maximal PPI (BID dosing) therapy, and in anyone exhibiting "red flag" signs or symptoms concerning for occult gastrointestinal malignancy.

4. A "step up" or "step down" approach to GERD treatment and maintenance is advocated at the lowest effective dose for acid suppression.

5. Reflux surgery is ideal for patients who respond to medical therapy and cannot tolerate adverse effects of medications, have a predominance of regurgitation, and are young and healthy and do not wish to continue long-term medication use.

# Key References

1. Kahrilas PJ, Shaheen NJ, Vaezi MF, et al; American Gastroenterological Association. American Gastroenterological Association Medical Position Statement on the management of gastroesophageal reflux disease. *Gastroenterology.* 2008;135(4):1383-1391.
2. Richter JE, Friedenberg FK. Gastroesophageal reflux disease. In: Feldman M, Friedman LS, Brandt LJ, eds. *Sleisenger and Fordtran's Gastrointestinal and Liver Disease: Pathophysiology/Diagnosis/Management.* Philadelphia, PA: Saunders Elsevier; 2010:705-726.

# CHAPTER 3

# DYSPHAGIA

MARK OVSIOWITZ, MD

*Dysphagia* is a general term that refers to the symptom of "difficult swallowing." Dysphagia can include difficulty with liquids, solids, or both. Although there are a vast number of causes of dysphagia, they generally can be classified into 2 main categories: oropharyngeal dysphagia and esophageal dysphagia. Oropharyngeal dysphagia refers to symptoms in which the underlying etiology is related to a problem with the mechanism or process of transferring food/liquid from the oropharyngeal cavity into the esophagus. Esophageal dysphagia refers to symptoms in which the underlying etiology is related to a problem with the esophagus itself or the lower esophageal sphincter. Esophageal dysphagia will be the focus of this chapter. The underlying causes can be broadly separated into two main categories: mechanical/anatomical causes or motility disorders. There are different diagnostic modalities used depending on which category is suspected. Therefore, a detailed history is of paramount importance. Some questions to focus on when conducting a dysphagia history include the following: symptoms with liquids versus solids versus both, intermittent or constant symptoms, progressive or stable symptoms, other underlying disease processes, other associated symptoms (eg, heartburn, weight loss, hematemesis), and a medication history.

Esrailian E. Gut Instincts: A Clinician's Handbook
of Digestive and Liver Diseases (pp 17-22).
© 2012 Taylor & Francis Group

# Diagnosis

Along with a detailed history, there are a number of diagnostic modalities that are useful in the evaluation of dysphagia. A barium esophagram is a noninvasive way of evaluating and imaging the esophagus. It does have some limitations and does not allow for tissue sampling or therapeutic interventions. However, it may be more sensitive than endoscopy in the evaluation of the proximal esophagus. Esophagogastroduodenoscopy (EGD) is another method available for the evaluation of dysphagia. It is very sensitive for the evaluation of structural lesions and allows for diagnostic sampling and therapeutic intervention. For these reasons, it is often the first test utilized. Figure 3-1 describes different diagnoses to consider after EGD, which is not useful for evaluating the function or motility of the esophagus. When it comes to these aspects, an esophageal manometry is the test of choice. Esophageal manometry should be used when an underlying motility disorder is suspected as the cause of dysphagia.

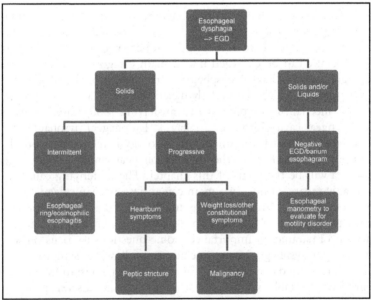

**Figure 3-1.** Possible etiologies for esophageal dysphagia. The workup will often begin with EGD if clinically appropriate.

# Common Diagnoses

## EOSINOPHILIC ESOPHAGITIS

Initially, eosinophilic esophagitis was thought to predominantly affect the pediatric and young adolescent population. However, over the years, it has been identified as a significant cause of dysphagia and food impaction in the adult population as well. Typically, patients will describe a history of intermittent dysphagia or food impactions. On some occasions, the initial presentation is in the emergency department as an acute impaction. Under normal conditions, eosinophils are absent in the esophageal mucosa. Eosinophilic esophagitis refers to a condition in which there is infiltration of eosinophils in the esophagus. Often, there is an association with allergies or asthma. The diagnosis of this condition requires EGD with esophageal biopsies. The typically described endoscopic findings include multiple esophageal rings, small esophageal plaques, linear furrows of the esophagus, and strictures. However, there are times when the endoscopic appearance is normal. To definitively make the diagnosis, esophageal biopsies must demonstrate an increased number of eosinophils. Although there is some debate over the exact number, 15 or more eosinophils per high-powered field is a commonly used cutoff. There also can be some overlap between eosinophilic esophagitis and gastroesophageal reflux disease (GERD) because reflux can also cause increased numbers of eosinophils in the esophagus. It is important to obtain multiple biopsies at different levels of the esophagus and keep them separated by level. GERD tends to affect the distal esophagus more predominantly than the proximal esophagus. Eosinophilic esophagitis does not have this same predisposition.

There are a few different approaches to therapy in patients with eosinophilic esophagitis. The first-line medical treatment usually includes swallowed topical fluticasone. Montelukast has also been used for treatment and maintenance. Elimination diets have also been used because of the association with allergies in some patients. In select situations, esophageal dilation may be required. Dilation should be done with extreme caution as the risk of perforation is substantially increased.

## PEPTIC STRICTURES

A peptic stricture refers to a narrowing of the esophagus that can occur as a result of exposure of the esophageal mucosa to acid. The most common of these conditions is GERD. Although a long history of heartburn symptoms is considered a risk factor, only a minority of patients with chronic GERD will ultimately develop peptic strictures. Dysphagia associated with a peptic stricture is usually progressive in nature. Initially, there may be difficulty swallowing solids. As the stricture worsens and the esophageal lumen becomes narrower, patients will begin to describe difficulty swallowing liquids. The time course for this progression is widely variable. Peptic strictures can be identified by barium study or EGD. Symptomatic peptic strictures can be dilated at the time of EGD. Depending on the severity of the stricture, serial dilations are sometimes required. Additionally, efforts to control the underlying GERD with medical management, such as proton pump inhibitor therapy, should be made.

## SCHATZKI'S RING

This is a benign mucosal ring that occurs at the gastroesophageal junction. The underlying etiology has not been defined clearly. However, there may be an association with GERD. Dysphagia caused by a Schatzki's ring usually involves solids and is intermittent in nature. These are best diagnosed during barium study or EGD when the esophagus is significantly distended. Symptomatic Schatzki's rings can be dilated at the time of EGD and usually with good long-term relief of symptoms.

## MALIGNANCY

Dysphagia secondary to esophageal cancer is generally the result of the mass effect and subsequent narrowing of the esophageal lumen. Therefore, the histologic type of cancer cannot be distinguished based on symptoms. Usually, the dysphagia is initially to solid foods. As the cancer grows and there is further luminal narrowing, the dysphagia may progress to involve liquids. There are often other constitutional symptoms of malignancy, such as weight loss. These mass lesions can be visualized by barium esophagram and EGD. The advantage of EGD is that it allows for biopsy samples to be obtained for confirmation of the diagnosis.

## MOTILITY DISORDERS

This broad category of disorders refers to the underlying function of the esophagus and/or esophageal sphincter. The dysphasia associated with motility disorders is usually to both solids and liquids. The diagnostic test of choice is esophageal manometry to measure the pressures and coordinated function of the esophagus and its sphincters. Some common examples of these disorders include achalasia, diffuse esophageal spasm, and nutcracker esophagus. The specifics of common motility disorders will be described in Chapter 4.

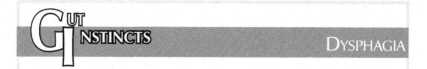

1. The underlying causes of esophageal dysphagia can be broadly separated into 2 main categories: mechanical/anatomical causes or motility disorders.

2. Eosinophilic esophagitis refers to a condition in which there is infiltration of eosinophils in the esophagus and requires biopsy to diagnose (usually ≥15 eosinophils per high-powered field).

3. Peptic strictures can be identified by barium study or EGD and can be dilated at the time of EGD.

4. Dysphagia caused by Schatzki's rings usually involves solids and is intermittent in nature.

5. The diagnostic test of choice for diagnosing esophageal motility disorders is esophageal manometry.

## Key References

1. Spechler SJ. AGA technical review on treatment of patients with dysphagia caused by benign disorders of the distal esophagus. *Gastroenterology*. 1999;117(1):233-254.

2. Kapel RC, Miller JK, Torres T, Aksoy S, Lash R, Katzka D. Eosinophilic esophagitis: a prevalent disease in the United States that affects all age groups. *Gastroenterology*. 2008;134(5):1316-1321.

# MOTILITY DISORDERS OF THE UPPER GASTROINTESTINAL TRACT

Jeffrey L. Conklin, MD, FACG

## Disorders of Esophageal Motor Function

The hallmark feature of disordered esophageal motor function is dysphagia sensed as food sticking at the suprasternal notch or substernally. Where it is sensed does not predict the location of the obstruction. Esophageal dysphagia is often sensed a few seconds after initiating the swallow. The disease processes that cause esophageal dysphagia and disordered esophageal function are detailed in Table 4-1. Painful swallowing (odynophagia) usually indicates a prominent inflammatory process like an esophageal ulcer. High-resolution esophageal pressure topographic manometry (HREPT) has allowed for better classification of these disorders.

## Achalasia

PRESENTATION

Achalasia is the best understood of all esophageal motor disorders. Pathophysiologically, it is a neuropathy of the myenteric plexus. The symptomatic hallmarks of achalasia are dysphagia when swallowing solids or liquids and chest pain. The dysphagia may be sensed substernally or at the suprasternal notch, and the chest pain often mimics coronary ischemia. The chest discomfort may also be felt as heartburn caused

Esrailian E. *Gut Instincts: A Clinician's Handbook
of Digestive and Liver Diseases* (pp 23-34).
© 2012 Taylor & Francis Group

| TABLE 4-1 | CAUSES OF DYSPHAGIA |
|---|---|
| **Dysphagia From the Pharynx and Striated Muscle Esophagus** | |
| Structural abnormalities | • Neoplasms (squamous cell cancer, lymphoma)<br>• Cricopharyngeal bar, Zenker's diverticulum<br>• Upper esophageal rings or webs (Plummer-Vinson syndrome)<br>• Extramural compression<br>  o Goiter, cervical vertebral osteophytes, dysphagia lusoria, lymph nodes |
| Neuro-muscular diseases | • Myopathic diseases<br>  o Muscular dystrophies (occulopharyngeal muscular dystrophy)<br>  o Polymyositis, dermatomyositis, inclusion body myositis<br>  o Metabolic myopathy (myxedema, thyrotoxicosis, steroid-induced myopathy)<br>• Diseases of the central nervous system<br>  o Cerebrovascular accident<br>  o Brainstem tumors<br>  o Bell's palsey<br>  o Parkinson's disease<br>  o Amyotrophic lateral sclerosis<br>  o Dementia<br>• Diseases of the peripheral nervous system<br>  o Myasthenia gravis<br>  o Poliomyelitis<br>  o Peripheral neuropathies (diabetes) |
| Other causes | • Infection<br>  o Candida<br>  o Cytomegalovirus (CMV)<br>  o Herpes simplex virus<br>• Surgery<br>  o Anterior surgical spine<br>  o Carotid endarterectomy<br>  o Thyroid, head, and neck resections<br>• Xerostomia<br>  o Sjogren's syndrome<br>• Medications<br>  o Anticholinergics<br>  o Antihistamines<br>  o Some antihypertensives |

*(continued)*

| TABLE 4-1 | CAUSES OF DYSPHAGIA (CONTINUED) |
|---|---|
| **Dysphagia From the Pharynx and Striated Muscle Esophagus** | |
| Other causes | • Radiation injury<br>• Medications<br>• Drugs affecting the central nervous system (CNS)<br>  o Sedatives<br>  o Anticonvulsants<br>  o Neuroleptics<br>  o Barbiturates<br>• Drugs affecting the peripheral nervous system (PNS)<br>  o Anticholinergics<br>  o Corticosteroids<br>  o L-tryptophan |
| **Dysphagia From the Smooth Muscle Esophagus** | |
| Mechanical obstruction | • Carcinoma of the esophagus or gastric cardia<br>• Intramural tumor (leiomyoma)<br>• Eosinophilic esophagitis<br>• Peptic stricture<br>• Foreign body<br>• Paraesophageal hernia<br>• Vascular compression (dysphagia aortica, left atrial enlargement)<br>• Mediastinal tumors<br>• Esophageal diverticula |
| Inflammatory | • Peptic esophagitis<br>• Infectious esophagitis (candida, CMV, herpes)<br>• Pill esophagitis<br>• Eosinophilic esophagitis<br>• Graft versus host disease<br>• Pemphigus/pemphigoid |
| Other causes | • Myopathic diseases (as above)<br>• CNS and PNS diseases<br>  o Parkinson's disease<br>  o Myasthenia gravis<br>  o Diabetes mellitus<br>• Primary motor disorders<br>  o Achalasia<br>  o Diffuse esophageal spasm<br>  o Hypotensive peristalsis |

*(continued)*

| TABLE 4-1 | CAUSES OF DYSPHAGIA (CONTINUED) |
|---|---|
| **Dysphagia From the Smooth Muscle Esophagus** | |
| Other causes | • Paraneoplastic syndrome (pseudoachalasia)<br>• Collagen vascular diseases (scleroderma)<br>• Hypothyroidism<br>• Amyloidosis<br>• Surgery<br>  o Nissen fundoplication<br>  o Laparoscopic band<br>  o Anastomotic strictures (gastric bypass, esophagectomy) |

by esophageal distention or fermentation of intraesophageal contents. Regurgitation of previously eaten food or a clear "slimy" or "bubbly" material (saliva) suggests esophageal obstruction. Early on, achalasia manifests primarily as dysphagia and chest pain, but these symptoms may fade with time. In its end stage, patients often report cough and regurgitation, particularly at night. These symptoms suggest the esophagus is greatly dilated and is acting as a reservoir.

## DIAGNOSIS

The diagnosis is made with esophagastroduodenoscopy (EGD), esophageal manometry, and the timed barium swallow. The endoscopic features of achalasia, while typical, are not diagnostic. They are food or bubbly saliva retained in the esophagus, esophageal dilation, and a tight gastroesophageal junction (EGJ) that takes some effort to pass. An upper endoscopy is needed to rule out intraluminal neoplasms of the esophagus or gastric cardia that can mimic achalasia. The timed barium swallow shows failure of esophageal peristalsis or uncoordinated motor activity, a "birds beak" configuration of the EGJ with failure of lower esophageal sphincter (LES) opening, and poor emptying of barium into the stomach. Esophageal manometry is the preferred test for diagnosing achalasia. The manometric features are failed or compromised LES relaxation and failure of peristalsis in the smooth muscle esophagus. When achalasia is diagnosed in the later decades of life, pseudoachalasia must be considered. Pseudoachalasia, which mimics achalasia clinically, is caused by neoplastic infiltration of the EGJ, or presumed humoral substances produced by a distant neoplasm, most notably small-cell cancer of the lung. In this setting, consideration should be given to getting CT scans of the chest and abdomen, endoscopic ultrasound, and a paraneoplastic panel.

## TREATMENT

Achalasia is the most treatable of esophageal motor disorders. It can be treated with botulinum toxin injection (100 to 200 IU) into the LES, large diameter (30 to 40 mm) balloon dilation of the EGJ, or Heller myotomy. In general, the use of botulinum toxin injection should be limited to patients who cannot tolerate other therapies because the effect of botulinum toxin wanes over time, necessitating repeated injections and, ultimately, it becomes ineffective when the immune system recognizes the toxin as a foreign protein. In addition, repeated injections cause scarring around the EGJ, making myotomy more difficult. Balloon dilation and Heller myotomy are both efficacious treatments, so the choice of therapy depends somewhat on local expertise.

# Functional Gastroesophageal Junction Obstruction

Functional EGJ obstruction manifests clinically as dysphagia and is diagnosed with HREPT. It is seen manometrically as an abnormally high pressure within the swallowed bolus as it is pushed down the esophagus ahead of a normal peristaltic contraction. In essence, it indicates obstruction to flow across the EGJ. Entities known to produce functional EGJ obstruction include fundoplication, peptic stricture, and eosinophilic esophagitis. On rare occasions, it may represent a variant of achalasia. Appropriate treatment depends on identifying the etiology of obstruction.

# Esophageal Spasm

## PRESENTATION

The spastic esophageal disorder traditionally called diffuse esophageal spasm (DES) presents clinically as dysphagia to solids and/or liquids that is substernal or at the suprasternal notch, and chest pain that may mimic cardiac ischemia. Eating or drinking something cold may precipitate the dysphagia and pain. Frequently, the patient says the pain comes on and is excruciating when something "gets stuck" in the esophagus. Some of these patients complain of heartburn that results either from true gastroesophageal reflux (GER) or muscle contraction that is sensed as heartburn.

## DIAGNOSIS

Endoscopy is always indicated in these patients to rule out neoplasm or inflammation as the cause of symptoms. The esophagus may take on a corkscrew appearance or contract in a random way. While suggestive, these findings are not diagnostic of DES. If the esophageal mucosa appears normal, mucosal biopsies should be taken to identify reflux esophagitis or eosinophilic esophagitis. A corkscrew pattern and/or chaotic contractile activity may also be seen with a barium swallow. Esophageal spasm is now subclassified based on the HREPT pattern. To diagnose spasm, at least 20% of wet swallows must generate contractions in the smooth muscle esophagus that propagate at a velocity of >8 cm$^{-1}$, which is indicative of a simultaneous contraction. The spasm is classified as diffuse if the entire smooth muscle esophagus is involved and segmental if only the proximal or distal half is involved.

## TREATMENT

Treatment of spastic esophageal disorders is somewhat of a hit-or-miss proposition. Several medical therapies have been successful anecdotally, but few are of proven benefit. Empiric treatment with proton pump inhibitors is reasonable, as GER is occasionally the cause of symptoms. Agents that inhibit smooth muscle contraction, such as nitrates, calcium channel antagonists, and type 5 phosphodiesterase inhibitors, decrease the amplitude of spastic contractions, but do not reliably treat the pain associated with esophageal spasm. Theophylline, a nonspecific phosphodiesterase inhibitor and adenosine receptor antagonist, has been used successfully to treat noncardiac chest pain. As with achalasia, injecting botulinum toxin into the smooth muscle esophagus sometimes transiently improves the symptoms of esophageal spasm. Low doses of trazodone or tricyclic antidepressants taken at night are efficacious treatment for esophageal pain. Other modulators of sensory pathways like pregabalin or gabapentin sometimes successfully attenuate esophageal pain. An infrequently used, but safe and sometimes effective therapy is baker's peppermint oil. It may require a bit of a mix-and-match approach with several of these medical options to successfully treat symptoms of esophageal spasm. Finally, a surgical approach, long esophageal myotomy, has been a proven and effective treatment for spasm.

# Hypertensive Peristalsis (Nutcracker Esophagus)

## Presentation

The typical clinical manifestations of hypertensive peristalsis are chest pain and, less commonly, dysphagia. These patients may also complain of heartburn that results either from GER or powerful esophageal contraction sensed as burning. Up to 50% of these patients have reflux esophagitis.

## Diagnosis

Although endoscopy is indicated to rule out esophageal cancer, it is characteristically normal. Mucosal biopsies should be obtained to look for reflux or eosinophilic esophagitis. Barium swallow is typically normal. Hypertensive peristalsis is diagnosed by manometry. Its manometric signature is normally propagating peristalsis in the smooth muscle esophagus that is more powerful (higher amplitude) than normal. Resting LES pressure and LES relaxation are normal.

## Treatment

Hypertensive peristalsis is for all practical purposes treated as a spastic esophageal disorder. Treatment for GER should be tried because many of these patients have reflux esophagitis. Modulators of pain pathways may also be of benefit.

# Aperistalsis (Absent Peristalsis) or Hypotensive Peristalsis in the Smooth Muscle Esophagus

## Presentation

Patients with either weak or no peristalsis in the smooth muscle esophagus frequently complain of dysphagia because the swallowed bolus is not easily transported. They may also complain of heartburn because gastric content refluxed into the esophagus is not adequately cleared back into the stomach.

## Diagnosis

While endoscopy is a useful way to identify esophageal inflammation or mechanical lesions causing dysphagia, it cannot diagnose disordered esophageal motor function. Nonetheless, finding bubbly saliva coating the esophageal wall suggests a problem with esophageal clearance.

The barium swallow does identify aperistalsis, but may not distinguish hypotensive from normal peristalsis. Weak peristalsis may leave part of the barium bolus behind in the esophageal lumen. Aperistalsis and hypotensive peristalsis are easily identified with esophageal manometry. Aperistalsis is the absence of a propagating peristaltic contraction in the smooth muscle esophagus. Hypotensive peristalsis is a normally propagating contraction that has an amplitude of less than 30 mm Hg over all or a significant portion (>3 cm) of the smooth muscle esophagus. Aperistalsis and hypotensive peristalsis are often associated with hypothyroidism, diabetes mellitus, or collagen vascular diseases (scleroderma). Amyloidosis, Parkinson's disease, myopathic diseases, or myasthenia gravis are less common causes.

## TREATMENT

There is little in the way of treatment for these "hypotensive" esophageal disorders. Identifying and treating those underlying pathological processes listed above may be of some benefit. Occasionally, esophageal motor function improves with the treatment of underlying reflux esophagitis. There is some experimental evidence that cholinergic agonists may improve poor esophageal motor function. This approach cannot be generally recommended as yet because it has not been adequately studied.

# Disorders of Pharyngeal and Upper Esophageal Sphincter Function

## PRESENTATION

Patients with abnormalities of pharyngeal motor function complain of dysphagia that is felt as food sticking high in the neck almost immediately upon swallowing. They may also complain of difficulty controlling food in the mouth, trouble starting the swallow, choking or coughing while eating, or nasopharyngeal reflux. They may have a "gurgly" or "wet" voice after eating, and their inability to protect the airway may lead to aspiration pneumonia. Malnutrition and dehydration may complicate their clinical course. The neuromuscular and structural abnormalities that cause these symptoms are reviewed in Table 4-1.

## DIAGNOSIS

Upper gastrointestinal endoscopy is of little value in the diagnosis of structural or functional abnormalities of the pharynx and upper esophageal sphincter function (UES). The cine-swallowing study or modified barium swallow with liquids and solids is the best way to examine complex pharyngeal motor processes during swallowing. It is essential for evaluating oropharyngeal dysphagia. Weak or uncoordinated pharyngeal contractions leave residue in the vallecullae or pyriform sinuses. A cricopharyngeal bar is seen as a prominent cricopharyngeus muscle and incomplete opening of the UES with swallowing. It also identifies aspiration, and dysfunction of the tongue and soft palate. The advent of HREPT makes manometric evaluation of the striated muscle components of the swallowing apparatus reliable for the first time. Elevated intrabolus pressure in the pharynx is a feature of either pharyngeal motor dysfunction or a cricopharyngeal bar obstructing flow across the UES. Weak or failed peristaltic contractions of the pharynx and striated muscle esophagus are easily identified.

## TREATMENT

The management of most pharyngeal motor problems is difficult. Speech pathologists may help by teaching safe swallowing techniques, and pharyngeal strengthening exercises are sometimes helpful. The cricopharyngeal bar can be successfully treated with dilation techniques or myotomy.

# Gastroparesis

## PRESENTATION

Gastroparesis is defined as delayed gastric emptying in the absence of mechanical small bowel or gastric outlet obstruction. It is more prevalent in women and increases with age. It is often associated with diabetes mellitus, particularly when the blood glucose is out of control or when there is diabetic neuropathy. Idiopathic cases often follow a viral gastroenteritis (postinfectious gastroparesis). It is occasionally a consequence of surgery, during which purposeful or inadvertent vagotomy occurred. It is less frequently associated with Parkinson's disease, collagen vascular diseases, amyloidosis, or intestinal pseudo-obstruction. No single etiology accounts for more than one-third of patients with gastroparesis.

The hallmark symptoms of gastroparesis are nausea, vomiting, early satiety, and bloating. It is also associated with abdominal pains of several types. The physical exam is usually nondescript. When fluid is retained in the stomach, a succussion splash may be elicited. A careful drug history should be obtained to identify the use of narcotic analgesics or other drugs that slow gastric emptying. It is important to remember that CNS processes that increase intracranial pressure cause nausea and vomiting. Finally, pregnancy should always be ruled out before embarking on a diagnostic workup using radiological procedures.

## DIAGNOSIS

Imaging of the stomach and small bowel (upper gastrointestinal [GI] series with small bowel follow-through, computed tomography [CT], or magnetic resonance [MR] enterography) and upper GI endoscopy are essential to rule out small bowel or gastric outlet obstruction before entertaining the diagnosis of gastroparesis. The diagnostic test of choice once obstructing lesions are ruled out is the scintigraphic gastric emptying study. A standard meal of toast, jam, and EggBeaters (ConAgra Foods, Omaha, NE) labeled with $^{99m}$Tc-sulfur colloid is eaten, and gastric retention is measured at 1, 2, and 4 hours. Gastric retention of more than 60% at 2 hours and more than 10% at 4 hours is consistent with gastroparesis. Other techniques including a $^{13}CO_2$ breath test, radiotelemetry capsule that measures pH, and ultrasound have been used to evaluate gastric emptying, but are not widely adopted in practice. Very specialized techniques like electrogastrography and antroduodenal manometry are available at specialized centers but are of little clinical utility in most cases.

## TREATMENT

The treatment of gastroparesis is tripartite: nutritional management, symptom reduction, and removal of aggravating factors. The dietary management of gastroparesis is extremely important. It should include small frequent meals that are low in fat and residue. The food may have to be soft, pureed, or even liquid. If the patient is unable to tolerate oral feeding, he or she can be managed with jejunostomy feeding or total parenteral nutrition.

A number of metabolic problems can exacerbate gastric emptying problems. Glucose control is extremely important in diabetic patients because blood glucose levels above 170 mg/dL slow gastric emptying. All patients, and especially diabetics, should be evaluated for hypothyroidism. When symptoms worsen acutely, electrolyte abnormalities, underlying infections, and diabetic ketoacidosis must be ruled out. Narcotic analgesics, calcium channel antagonists, nitrates, phosphodiesterase inhibitors, and drugs with anticholinergic activity can slow gastric emptying.

Patients with gastroparesis often have more generalized disorders of gastrointestinal motor function that predispose them to small intestinal bacterial overgrowth (SIBO). These patients typically complain of bloating, gas, and abdominal distention. It can be diagnosed with a lactulose or glucose hydrogen breath test, or it can be treated empirically with antibiotics. Rifaxamin, a nonabsorbable rifamycin analogue given 400 to 550 mg, 3 times daily for 10 to 14 days, is the most effective therapy for SIBO.

A number of agents can be used to treat the nausea of gastroparesis. They include phenothiazines (promethazine, prochloperazine), dopamine agonists (metoclopramide 10 mg, 4 times daily; domperidone 20 mg, 4 times daily), serotonin 3 receptor antagonist (ondansetron 4 to 8 mg, 3 times daily), and a cannabinoid (dronabinol 5 to 10 mg, twice daily). Unfortunately, metoclopramide has a neurological side effect profile that limits its use, and domperidone requires an Investigational New Drug and Institutional Review Board approval. Although metoclopramide and domperidone are touted as promotility agents, they have little effect on gastric emptying. Erythromycin (2 to 3 mg/kg, 3 times daily), acting as a motilin analogue, does have promotility activity. It triggers phase 3 of the migration myoelectrical complex, which sweeps undigestible materials from the stomach and small intestine. Care must be taken with its use because it has been linked to sudden cardiac death caused by prolonging the QT interval syndrome. It is most effective when given intravenously, and its efficacy wanes rapidly due to tachyphalaxis. Another macrolide antibiotic, azithromycin, also has promotility activity and is not linked to the prolonged QT syndrome. Its efficacy is now being evaluated. Adequate control of nausea may require using more than one class of drug simultaneously. Medications formulated as liquids or suppositories may be most useful.

Why patients with gastroparesis have abdominal pain is not entirely known. Agents that modulate pain pathways are often beneficial. Narcotic analgesics may be needed, but they must be used judiciously.

The FDA has not yet approved gastric electrical stimulation (GES) to treat gastroparesis, but its usefulness has been demonstrated anecdotally and in clinical trials. GES improves nausea and vomiting but does not accelerate gastric emptying. The key to its efficacy is appropriate patient selection. Success is most likely in patients with diabetes and when the predominant symptoms are nausea and vomiting. It is important to maintain good diabetic control for the reasons outlined above. Predictors of failure include idiopathic gastroparesis, abdominal pain, narcotic use, and/or psychiatric illness. Today, GES should be undertaken only at centers with special expertise in its use.

Injecting botulinum toxin into the pylorus has been used, with the rationale that it should relax the pylorus as it does the lower esophageal sphincter. This approach is controversial because its efficacy is uncertain. Having said this, it can be remarkably effective in selected patients and is safe.

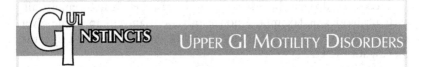

**G**UT**I**NSTINCTS    UPPER GI MOTILITY DISORDERS

1. Dysphagia is an alarm symptom that requires careful evaluation to rule out esophageal neoplasms.
2. The diagnostic features of achalasia are failure of lower esophageal sphincter relaxation and failure of peristalsis in the smooth muscle esophagus.
3. Treatment of achalasia with botulinum toxin should be reserved for patients unable to tolerate large-caliber balloon dilation or Heller myotomy.
4. The diagnosis of gastroparesis should be made only after small bowel obstruction and pyloric stenosis have been ruled out.
5. The treatment of gastroparesis is complicated and includes careful nutritional management, symptom reduction, and removal of aggravating factors.

## Key References

1. Conklin JL, Pimentel M, Soffer E, eds. *Color Atlas of High-Resolution Manometry.* New York, NY: Springer Science and Business Media LLC; 2009.
2. Hasler WL. Gastroparesis: Symptoms, evaluation and treatment. *Gastroenterol Clin North Am.* 2007;36(3):619-647, ix.
3. Kahrilas PJ, Smout JPM. Esophageal disorders. *Am J Gastroenterol.* 2010;105(4):747-756.
4. Spechler JS. AGA technical review on treatment of patients with dysphagia caused by benign disorders of the distal esophagus. *Gastroenterology.* 1999;117(1):233-254.

# CHAPTER 5

# BARRETT'S ESOPHAGUS

Bennett E. Roth, MD

Barrett's esophagus (BE) is defined as the metaplastic replacement of the squamous esophageal mucosal surface by intestinalized columnar mucosa. Although originally inclusive of any columnar mucosal changes in the esophagus, it is only that associated with intestinalization (intestinal metaplasia) of the columnar cells that carries the risk of cancer and should be considered Barrett's mucosa. Intestinal metaplasia can occur in the gastric cardia and must be distinguished from that arising in the true esophagus because the former, which may be a marker for underlying gastroesophageal reflux disease (GERD), is not associated with an increased risk for malignancy. Adenocarcinoma of the esophagus accounts for approximately 60% of all esophageal cancers and most often arises from underlying BE. However, the risk of developing cancer in those with known BE is approximately 0.5% annually with an overall lifetime risk of 1.5% to 2%.

## Epidemiology

The vast majority of BE is associated with underlying GERD. The true prevalence is unknown. GERD affects a large portion of the population, with more than 45% of Americans experiencing reflux at least monthly, and the majority of whom are not evaluated with endoscopy. However, BE is found in 3% of those undergoing endoscopy because of reflux symptoms and in 1% of those scoped for all reasons. BE is

Esrailian E. *Gut Instincts: A Clinician's Handbook of Digestive and Liver Diseases* (pp 35-40).
© 2012 Taylor & Francis Group

3 times more common in men, increases with age, and is far more common in Whites compared to Asians or African-Americans. Additional possible risk factors for BE include obesity and diets rich in animal fat. Diets high in fruits and vegetables seem to decrease the risk. There are conflicting data regarding the associations between alcohol and smoking and an increased risk of BE, as opposed to a clearer association in squamous carcinoma of the esophagus.

## Diagnosis

BE is a combined endoscopic and histologic diagnosis. The hallmarks of the endoscopic appearance are the irregular proximal migration of the salmon-colored mucosal surface (which is typical in the stomach) up into the true esophagus and/or the presence of focal "islands" above the squamocolumnar junction (Z line). BE is also subclassified into long and short segments (greater or less than 3 cm of involvement). It is critical that landmarks be determined at the time of biopsy. Confusion can occur in the setting of a hiatal hernia because under- or overinflation of the hernia may distort the true location of the esophagogastric junction. With appropriate air insufflation, the most proximal border of the gastric folds can be determined. This coincides with the true junctional area and can be used to distinguish gastric from esophageal biopsies. Only the finding of intestinal metaplasia within the true esophagus defines the presence of BE. Care must be taken to avoid biopsies in areas of ulceration because inflammation may mask the presence of intestinal metaplasia and cause difficulty in the diagnosis of dysplasia. Therefore, it is wise to treat underlying GERD for at least 6 weeks prior to endoscopy if searching for BE. Initial biopsies should be obtained at 4 quadrants from every 2 cm of visible BE as well as from isolated islands. In addition, irregular bumps or undulations of the mucosal surface should be biopsied, noted in the procedure report for location, and, if dysplasia is found, followed up with endoscopic ultrasound. If any evidence of dysplasia is documented, repeat endoscopic biopsies at 1-cm increments of all visible BE should be performed.

## Management of Barrett's Esophagus

In light of the association with GERD, all patients should be vigorously and continually treated with antisecretory medication. Although many promote the use of twice-daily treatment with proton pump inhibitors, there are no definitive studies proving the benefit of this approach. There is no evidence that BE can be significantly reversed with the use of acid inhibition. Once identified, patients must be enrolled in a regular surveillance protocol. In the absence of dysplasia on initial investigation, a repeat endoscopy with biopsies should be done at 1 year. If no dysplasia is encountered, repeat examinations are recommended every 3 years. There is growing evidence that this interval may be safely extended to 5 years.

If low-grade dysplasia (LGD) is found, repeat examinations are recommended yearly until there is none encountered or there is evidence of progression to high-grade dysplasia (HGD) or carcinoma. The finding of HGD sets into motion a series of options for further intervention. It is essential that experts in gastrointestinal pathology confirm the finding of HGD. Often, this requires review by additional pathologists. If HGD is confirmed with evidence of mucosal mass, undulation, or ulceration, endoscopic ultrasound (EUS) is recommended to search for evidence of invasive carcinoma. If this examination is normal, further options include repeat endoscopic surveillance at 3-month intervals, endoscopic ablation, endoscopic mucosal resection (EMR), or esophagectomy. The latter was the standard of care until recent years. However, during the past 5 to 10 years, endoscopic therapy has gained increased favor. A visible nodule without identified growth beyond the upper submucosa can be removed by EMR. The resected margin must be examined for absence of Barrett's mucosa to ensure complete resection. If there is BE (with or without dysplasia) still at the resection margin, by definition, the patient has an invasive carcinoma with risk of lymph node involvement as high as 20%. These individuals should be offered surgery in the absence of medical contraindications. If the resected nodule is completely excised, the remaining Barrett's mucosa can be treated with endoscopic ablative techniques. These include radiofrequency ablation, photodynamic therapy, cryotherapy, and/or endoscopic mucosal resection. Success rates for eradication of high-grade dysplasia are as high as 90% with complete eradication of Barrett's mucosa successfully achieved in more than 85% of cases. See Figure 5-1 for a summary of this approach.

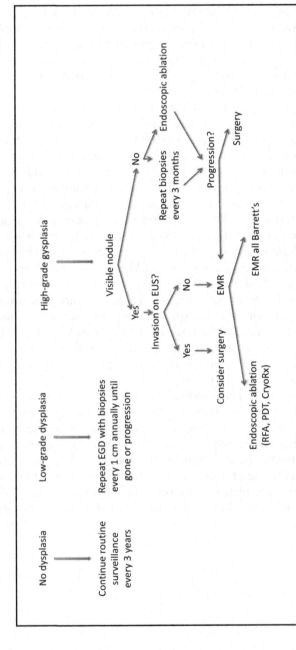

**Figure 5-1.** Management of dysplasia. (EUS indicates endoscopic ultrasound; EMR, endoscopic mucosal resection; RFA, radiofrequency ablation; PDT, photodynamic therapy; CryoRx, cryotherapy)

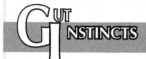

1. It is essential to document the location of endoscopic landmarks for biopsies to ensure proper interpretation and appropriate diagnosis of BE.
2. Although the risk of adenocarcinoma of the esophagus is higher in patients with BE, it is still quite low with an annual risk of no more than 0.5%.
3. Caucasian men older than 50, with a 5-year or more history of reflux disease, are the highest risk group for BE.
4. Continued surveillance at 3- to 5-year intervals is recommended for patients with Barrrett's in the absence of dysplasia.
5. The treatment of high-grade dysplasia is evolving away from surgery and toward less morbid endoscopic modalities.

## Key References

1. Wang KK, Sampliner RE. Updated guidelines 2008 for the diagnosis, surveillance and therapy of Barrett's esophagus. *Am J Gastroenterol.* 2008;103(3): 788-797.
2. Sikkmea M, de Jonge PJ, Steyerberg EW, Kuipers EJ. Risk of esophageal adenocarcinoma and mortality in patients with Barrett's esophagus: a systematic review and meta-analysis. *Clin Gastroenterol Hepatol.* 2010;8(3):235-244.
3. Spechler S, Fitzgerald RC, Prasad GA, Wang KK. History, molecular mechanisms, and endoscopic treatment of Barrett's esophagus. *Gastroenterol.* 2010;138(3):854-869.

CHAPTER

# 6

# Upper Gastrointestinal Tract Malignancies

Zev A. Wainberg, MD, MSc

Malignancies of the upper gastrointestinal (GI) tract can be divided anatomically based on the location: esophagus (proximal or distal), gastroesophageal junction (GEJ), or stomach. These diseases can also be divided pathologically: squamous cell cancer of the esophagus, adenocarcinoma of the GEJ, and adenocarcinoma of the stomach. Although all of these diseases may arise from the upper GI tract, they are heterogeneous in their clinical behavior. For patients in the United States without either a family history or genetic predisposition, there are no screening recommendations for cancers of the upper GI tract. In contrast, in Asia where the incidence of these diseases is so much higher, screening of gastric and esophageal cancers is established as the standard of care.

## Esophageal Cancer

### Squamous Cell Carcinoma

Squamous cell carcinoma (SCC) occurs most often in the proximal two-thirds of the esophagus. Although this cancer has decreased in incidence in the United States, it is still the most prevalent histologic subtype in the world. SCC of the esophagus has been linked to tobacco smoking and/or excessive alcohol abuse. Cigarette smoking and alcohol

Esrailian E. *Gut Instincts: A Clinician's Handbook of Digestive and Liver Diseases* (pp 41-46).
© 2012 Taylor & Francis Group

appear to act synergistically, thus producing high relative risks in heavy users of cigarettes and alcohol.

### ADENOCARCINOMA

This histologic subtype of esophagus cancer most commonly occurs in the distal esophagus and GEJ. During the past 30 years, it has become much more common than SCC of the esophagus. While smoking may be a risk factor for this subtype as well, alcohol has not been linked. Barrett's esophagus and gastroesophageal reflux disease (GERD) have emerged as risk factors for this disease.

## Diagnosis and Staging of Esophageal Cancer

Regardless of the subtype, esophagus cancers are diagnosed by endoscopy with biopsy. Staging is critical to determining the appropriate therapies. Endoscopic ultrasound (EUS) is both sensitive (>90%) and specific for establishing the depth of tumor invasion (T stage), but less accurate in determining nodal involvement (N stage). The role of fine needle aspiration (FNA) of lymph nodes by EUS is controversial.

Computed tomography (CT) scans of the chest, abdomen, and pelvis are mandatory to assess for both local involvement and, more importantly, the presence of distant metastasis. The pattern of metastasis is different between SCC and adenocarcinomas, with the former often having lung involvement and the latter involving more abdominal organs. Positron emission tomography (PET) scans have now been well-validated in improving both the sensitivity and specificity of staging and are now widely considered to be part of the standard of care. A bone scan should be considered if patients have bone pain or greatly elevated levels of alkaline phosphatase.

Unfortunately, only 40% to 50% of patients with esophagus cancer present with clinically localized disease. The 5-year survival is entirely stage dependent with more than 80% of patients diagnosed with Stage I disease (T1N0M0) having 5-year survival, 15% to 30% of those with Stage II to III (T2-T3, N0-N1) having 5-year survival, and less than 5% of those with Stage IV (metastasis) having 5-year survival.

## Treatment of Esophageal Cancer

### TREATMENT OF STAGE I DISEASE

Most people believe esophagectomy is the standard treatment for early esophagus cancers. The extent of surgical resection and type of procedure (Ivor-Lewis or transthoracic versus transhiatal) is still a matter of debate. Recently, less invasive procedures, such as endoscopic mucosal resection (EMR) and photodynamic therapy (PDT), have emerged as important tools in the treatment of early disease. However, at this time, for medically fit patients, they are not yet considered the standard of care.

## Treatment of Locally Advanced Disease

The management of patients with Stage II and III esophagus cancers is a matter of great controversy, and no consensus has emerged despite many years of research. The options for management include surgery and chemotherapy, surgery and chemoradiation, or chemotherapy and radiation. Based on several large randomized clinical trials, one thing is clear: radiation, chemotherapy, and surgery as stand-alone treatments are insufficient.

## Treatment of Advanced Disease

The goal of treatment under these circumstances is palliation, and palliative resection is almost never indicated. Local approaches such as radiation or esophageal stent placement could be considered as dictated by symptoms. Combination chemotherapies are the standard of care for these patients and have been shown to improve both overall survival and morbidity. Most practitioners consider fluoropyrimidine and platinum agents to be among the most active and the best choice for initial therapies. Other chemo agents with activity include the taxanes, camptothecins, and anthracyclines. Unfortunately, this treatment is entirely palliative, and the median overall survival despite recent improvements remains less than 1 year. Figure 6-1 outlines a treatment algorithm for the treatment of patients with esophagus cancer.

# Gastric Cancer

Gastric cancers are more common than esophageal cancer in the Western world, although their incidence is decreasing. This disease is defined as any malignant tumor arising from the GEJ to the pylorus, although tumors that arise from the GEJ are often classified as a separate entity. Globally, most cases of gastric cancer occur in Asia, and an association between diet and environment has been linked. Classic risk factors that have been linked to gastric cancer include intestinal metaplasia, previous gastric resection, pernicious anemia, family history, and infection with *Helicobacter pylori*. While the overall risk of developing gastric cancer in the presence of *H. pylori* infection is low, more than >40% of cases are linked with it. Unlike esophagus cancer, adenocarcinomas account for more than 95% of cases, and other subtypes (GI stromal tumors, lymphomas) are rare.

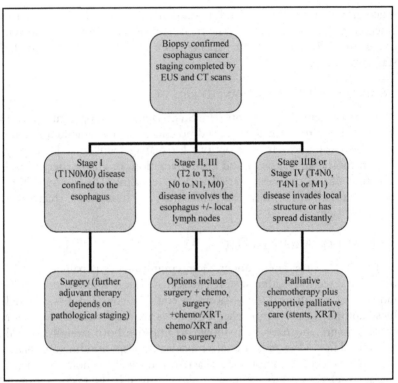

**Figure 6-1.** Diagnosis and treatment of esophagus cancer. (EUS indicates endoscopic ultrasound; XRT, radiation therapy; CT, computed tomography; TNM, staging system used for cancer.)

## DIAGNOSIS AND STAGING OF GASTRIC CANCER

Like esophagus cancers, most cases of gastric cancer are diagnosed at an advanced stage. The diagnosis is established endoscopically, and once it has been established, it is staged in much the same way as esophagus cancer. Computed tomography scans are critical to assess nodal involvement and metastatic spread but, unlike esophagus cancer, the role of PET scans in gastric cancer is not clearly established. Endoscopic ultrasound is also an important staging technique to assess depth of tumor invasion and perigastric nodal involvement. Laparoscopic staging is often indicated in this disease to detect small-volume visceral and peritoneal metastasis missed on CT scan.

# Treatment of Gastric Cancer

## TREATMENT OF STAGE I DISEASE

Management of early gastric cancer relies on surgical resection of the involved stomach with reconstruction to preserve intestinal continuity. The extent of resection depends on the site and extent of the primary tumor with a subtotal gastrectomy being the preferred approach. The extent of lymphadenectomy (D1 versus D2 dissections) has been the source of much investigation and remains an area of controversy. While improved long-term survival rates for Japanese patients have been attributed to the more aggressive D2 surgery, most surgeons in the Western world feel that the higher postoperative morbidity and mortality associated with this surgery does not warrant its routine use.

## TREATMENT OF LOCALLY ADVANCED DISEASE

For patients with locally advanced disease (Stage II to III), treatment is controversial. Based on recent randomized clinical trials, most practitioners advocate for neoadjuvant chemotherapy prior to surgery. An alternative to this approach is proceeding directly to surgery, and then treatment with either chemotherapy or chemoradiation can be considered adjuvantly.

## TREATMENT OF METASTATIC GASTRIC CANCER

As in esophagus cancer, the 5-year survival of patients with metastatic gastric cancer is less than 5%. Most clinical trials have combined these patients with patients with metastatic esophageal cancer, and as in that disease, the standard is combination therapy. The median survival is also approximately 9 to 12 months, and chemotherapy is given with palliative intent.

## Gut Instincts — UPPER GI TRACT MALIGNANCIES

1. Upper GI cancers are primarily classified into 3 groups: SCC of the esophagus, adenocarcinoma of the esophagus, and adenocarcinoma of the stomach.

2. Each group is associated with unique pathologic, epidemiologic, and treatment differences.

3. All patients should get accurately staged with computed tomography scans of the chest/abdomen/pelvis and endoscopic ultrasound.

4. Treatment and prognosis is stage dependent, and patients with early stage disease can undergo successful surgical cures.

5. Most patients present with advanced disease, and treatment is often palliative, consisting of chemotherapy and supportive care.

## Key References

1. Locke GR III, Talley NJ, Carpenter HA, Harmsen WS, Zinsmeister AR, Melton LJ III. Changes in the site- and histology-specific incidence of gastric cancer during a 50-year period. *Gastroenterology*. 1995;109(6):1750-1756.

2. Younes M, Henson DE, Ertan A, Miller CC. Incidence and survival trends of esophageal carcinoma in the United States: racial and gender differences by histological type. *Scand J Gastroenterol*. 2002;37(12):1359-1365.

3. Sarela AI, Lefkowitz R, Brennan MF, Karpeh MS. Selection of patients with gastric adenocarcinoma for laparoscopic staging. *Am J Surg*. 2006;191(1):134-138.

# 7

# NUTRITION

Leo Treyzon, MD, MS

Nutrition represents, for the gastroenterologist, what pharmaceuticals represent for the internist: an indispensable tool for the treatment of most gastrointestinal (GI) conditions. In an outpatient setting, 2 of the most common patient-driven nutritional concerns deal with the management of bloating and weight-loss efforts.

## Bloating

The differential diagnosis of bloating is broad and includes conditions such as lactose intolerance, fructose intolerance, small intestinal bacterial overgrowth, irritable bowel syndrome (IBS), constipation, diarrhea, dyspepsia, obesity, celiac disease, food hypersensitivity, and other disorders.

### DIETARY CONSIDERATIONS FOR TREATMENT OF BLOATING AND FLATULENCE

High gas-producing foods include beans, brussel sprouts, onions, cabbage, celery, raw carrots, raisins, prune juice, apricots, wheat germ, artificial sweeteners, and sugar alcohols. Moderately gas-producing foods include dairy (yogurt, milk, cheese), bananas, eggplant, bell peppers, cucumber skins, apples, broccoli, cauliflower, asparagus, high-fructose corn syrup, carbonated beverages, sugar-free gums, garlic, and

Esrailian E. *Gut Instincts: A Clinician's Handbook of Digestive and Liver Diseases* (pp 47-52).
© 2012 Taylor & Francis Group

fatty or fried foods. Low gas-producing foods, and thus usually well tolerated, include meat, poultry, fish, eggs, some vegetables in limited amounts (lettuce, tomato, avocado), some fruits (cherries, grapes, and cantaloupe), rice, pasta, oatmeal, corn chips, popcorn, and chocolate.

Patients bothered by bloating should try a 4-week gas-reducing diet. Improvement usually occurs early in 1 week. Subsequently, foods are reintroduced, and the patient learns to identify the offending meal components and to avoid them to prevent recurrence of gas. After the patient identifies an offending agent, he or she can decide whether the pleasure of the food is worth the price paid from consuming it subsequently. Low FODMAP (fermentable oligosaccharides, disaccharides, monosaccharides, and polyols) intake may significantly impact subjective bloating.

In general, it is preferred to eat 3 meals daily as opposed to grazing throughout the day. Creating an interdigestive rest period is more likely to stimulate the migrating motor complex (MMC) to ensure productive peristalsis and prevention of bacterial overgrowth.

# Obesity

Obesity is best characterized as excess adiposity. It is conveniently gauged best by the body mass index (BMI). Obesity is both a national and international epidemic. After smoking, it is the second most common cause of preventable death. In regards to gastroenterologists, deaths attributable to obesity far outnumber deaths attributable to colon cancer. Prevention appears to be the best treatment.

## TREATMENT OF OVERWEIGHT AND OBESE PATIENTS

Treatment options are based on the BMI, presence of weight-related comorbidities, and motivation of the patient to undergo weight loss efforts. Secondary causes of abnormal weight gain should be considered (Table 7-1). Diets, pharmacotherapy, and behavior modification with or without exercise are the available nonsurgical treatments. Diet therapy alone is the most commonly prescribed method. Using diet alone, weight loss at 1 year is modest, and likelihood of weight regain is more than 90%.

For most obese adults, exercise alone without caloric restriction barely yields appreciable changes in weight. The addition of mild to moderate exercise efforts to caloric restriction surprisingly also does not lead to clinically significant increases in weight loss. Exercise daily, however, appears to be of vital importance for maintenance of weight loss.

| TABLE 7-1 | SECONDARY CAUSES OF OBESITY AND ABNORMAL WEIGHT GAIN |
|---|---|
| **Cause** | **Comments** |
| Hypothalamic obesity | Watch for endocrine disturbance, impaired vision, excessive thirst, headaches, neurologic disturbances, or behavior changes |
| Medications | Corticosteroids, anti-psychotics, anti-depressants, anti-epileptics, antidiabetes medications |
| Cushing's syndrome | Dexamethasone suppression test |
| Hypogonadism | Screen with serum total testosterone |
| Polycystic ovary syndrome (PCOS) | Screen with luteinizing hormone and follicle-stimulating hormone |
| Hypothyroidism | Screen with thyroid-stimulating hormone and thyroid function tests |
| Sedentary lifestyle | Often occurs after a musculoskeletal injury or change to a new job |
| Menopause | Common |
| Psychiatric disturbances | Most common are depression and binge eating disorder |
| Smoking cessation | Common |
| Genetic obesity syndromes | Rare and usually identified in childhood (eg, Prader-Willi syndrome) |

The addition of pharmacotherapy to diet therapy is more efficacious than diet therapy alone. One diet drug that is approved in the United States for long-term weight loss is orlistat (Xenical, Genentech, San Francisco, CA). Cost and side effect profile somewhat limits the widespread use of this agent in common practice. Orlistat is known to cause diarrhea. Phentermine is a commonly used agent approved only for short-term weight loss efforts (<12 weeks), and it seems to suppress hunger. Patients often become tolerant to this medication, and higher doses are often not employed. Furthermore, long-term use may be associated with cardiovascular risks as well. Weight regain appears to be common to all these medications with cessation of use and discontinuation of dietary efforts. Table 7-2 details a simplified checklist for managing obesity that can be used by the practicing clinician.

| TABLE 7-2 | THE GASTROENTEROLOGIST'S SIMPLIFIED CHECKLIST FOR MANAGING OBESITY |
|-----------|-------------------------------------------------------------------|
| **To Do Item** | **Comments** |
| Assess motivation to lose weight | If not motivated to make efforts, it is better to set up strategies to prevent further weight gain. Do not start weight loss efforts, because patient will likely fail and become further frustrated. |
| Screen for secondary causes of obesity | See Table 7-1. |
| Perform basic history and physical exam | Attention to BMI, blood pressure, waist circumference, abdominal striae, glycogenic acanthosis, edema, arthropathy, oropharyngeal signs of sleep apnea. |
| Perform basic lab tests | CBC, fasting CMP, TSH, fasting lipid panel, EKG |
| Set start date and outline realistic weight goals | Schedule follow-up to ensure compliance at regular intervals (ie, monthly visits). |
| Define diet plan | Consider self-imposed caloric restriction, commercial programs like Weight Watchers (Weight Watchers International, New York, NY), or meal replacement plans like Nutrisystem (Nutrisystem, Inc, Fort Washington, PA). Offer dietetic consultation. |
| Give a weekly exercise prescription | First week can be as simple as going to the mailbox daily. Second week can be a 5-minute walk. Third week is a daily 10-minute walk. |
| Ensure adequate hydration | 64 oz of noncaloric beverages (good rule of thumb is to have clear or light yellow urine). Limit all caloric beverages (eg, coffee creamers, juices, and alcohol). |
| | *(continued)* |

| TABLE 7-2 | THE GASTROENTEROLOGIST'S SIMPLIFIED CHECKLIST FOR MANAGING OBESITY (CONTINUED) |
|---|---|
| **To Do Item** | **Comments** |
| Ensure adequate sleep | Goal is 8 hours of uninterrupted sleep. |
| Teach self-monitoring | Highlight importance of food journaling. Encourage patient to purchase a calorie counter handbook (low-cost) to estimate caloric values of foods. |
| Encourage behavioral modification curriculum | Recommend purchase of a patient-oriented book for self-education. The curriculum should highlight self-monitoring, stimulus control, cognitive restructuring, stress management, and social support. |

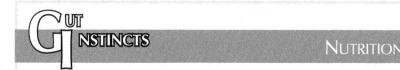

GUT INSTINCTS                    NUTRITION

1. Secondary causes of obesity are not common. Most often, patients develop excess weight due to inappropriate food intake and sedentary lifestyle, which is partly genetically predetermined.

2. Weight loss surgery is the treatment of choice for appropriately selected individuals who have a Class II obesity (BMI >35) with weight-related comorbid conditions, and patients with Class III obesity (BMI >40) with or without comorbid conditions.

3. Weight loss surgery is associated with reduced cardiovascular and other weight-related risks, reduced all-cause mortality, and reduced health care costs. This treatment is appropriate in selected individuals until such time when more effective weight loss treatments are developed.

4. More than 90% of self-directed weight loss efforts will ultimately fail. Patient monitoring in a formal program offers higher success rates.

5. Treatment of abdominal bloating is accomplished by avoidance of gas-producing foods and consumption of 3 meals daily. Fostering an interdigestive rest period of 4 to 5 hours creates stimulation of the MMC.

# Key References

1. Azpiroz F, Malagelada JR. Abdominal bloating. *Gastroenterology.* 2005; 129(3):1060-1078.
2. Bray, GA. *Contemporary Diagnosis and Management of Obesity.* 2nd ed. Newton, PA: Handbooks in Health Care, Co; 2003.

# FEEDING TUBES
## PLACEMENT AND MANAGEMENT
## FOR THE CLINICIAN

Stanley Dea, MD

## Nasogastric Tubes

Nasogastric (NG) tubes are often used as the initial route of enteral feedings. Although Salem Sump tubes (Covidien, Mansfield, MA) are commonly used for feedings, the risk of nasal irritation and sinusitis make them a poor choice for long-term feeding. Tubes specifically designed for feeding come in different lengths and sizes. The shorter (36-inch) and wider (16F) tubes are softer than Salem-Sump tubes but can still be uncomfortable. The longer (45-inch) small-bore (8F) tubes are more comfortable and can provide postpyloric or duodenal feeding for patients with gastroparesis. Patients who require long-term NG tube feeding should use a small-bore tube. Disadvantages of small-bore tubes include clogging and possible inadvertent placement in the lungs, making a postplacement x-ray necessary before starting feeding.

## Gastrostomy Tubes

Gastrostomy tubes (G-tubes) placed endoscopically are called percutaneous endoscopic gastrostomy (PEG) tubes. Advantages of PEG tubes include easy placement and the ability to insert at the bedside in the intensive care unit. Endoscopic visualization of the tube site in

Esrailian E. *Gut Instincts: A Clinician's Handbook of Digestive and Liver Diseases* (pp 53-58).
© 2012 Taylor & Francis Group

the stomach can make gastric tumors or ulcers visible prior to place-ment. Interventional radiology (IR) places tubes under fluoroscopy, but requires NG tube placement to insufflate the stomach prior to G-tube placement. This is useful if an endoscope cannot be passed into the stomach during PEG placement (eg, a near-obstructing esophageal cancer). A small-bore NG tube can be placed with subsequent IR place-ment of a gastrostomy tube. Disadvantages of IR-guided tube placement include the need for T-fasteners to hold the skin to the stomach wall and lack of direct visualization during placement. Surgical placement of tubes is usually done concomitantly with other surgical procedures.

Gastrostomy tubes have internal bumpers that keep them in place. The PEG tubes that are initially placed have a soft-retention dome that will deform when pulled on to allow traction removal at the bedside. Some tubes have a hard plastic bumper that cannot be removed by pull-ing on it. There are no numbers or markings on these tubes, which is a clue that it may not be able to be removed by traction. These tubes (and any tube not easily removed with traction) should be removed endoscopically. Most IR-placed tubes and G-tube replacements have a water-filled balloon at the end as a bumper. Similar to Foley catheters, balloon-type replacements can be easily removed and replaced by deflat-ing the balloon.

# Indications and Contraindications for Gastrostomy Tube Placement

The major indications for enteral feeding are aspiration risk (eg, post-stroke or neurologic condition), esophageal or oropharyngeal obstruc-tion (eg, cancer), and inability to feed (eg, coma, severe dementia).

Contraindications for gastrostomy tube placement include poor prognosis (eg, fewer than 3 months' survival), gastric ulcer or tumor obstructing the tube entry site, gastric outlet obstruction or severe gastroparesis, and technical problems (eg, prior resection or altered anatomy).

Prior to placing a gastrostomy tube, items to check include the following: patient's ability to tolerate NG tube feeding; any signs of systemic infection; aspirin, anti-platelet agent, or anticoagulant use; history of prior abdominal surgery; and PEG placement is elective, and consent must be obtained.

## Gastrostomy Tube Postplacement Care

Multiple studies have now confirmed that feedings can be started shortly after placement. Protocols have started feedings as early as 4 hours after placement with rapid advancement of feeding every 4 hours.

Residuals should be checked every 4 hours initially for continuous feeding or prior to every bolus feeding. Feedings should be held for 1 hour for residuals greater than 150 mL. If residuals are persistently high, prokinetic agents such as metoclopramide can be used, or feedings can be switched to a more concentrated form.

Feeding instructions should include raising the head of the bed 30 degrees to 45 degrees to reduce aspiration. Water (150 mL) should be flushed through the tube every 8 hours to prevent clogging and to add additional free water. Medicines should be given in liquid form with 100 mL of water flushed afterwards. If the G-tube site is clean without bleeding or weeping, no dressing is necessary. The site can be cleaned with soap and water.

# Troubleshooting Gastrostomy Tubes

## PEG PULLED OUT INADVERTENTLY

If tube placement was fewer than 2 weeks ago, do not replace the tube as the tract is immature. Placement of a G-tube replacement through an immature tract can lead to feeds entering the peritoneum with possible sepsis or death. Tubes from 2 to 4 weeks old can be replaced with caution, and use of fluoroscopic guidance is advised. Tracts more than 4 weeks old are considered mature, and tubes can be replaced at the bedside. If a tube is not readily available, a suitably sized Foley catheter can be placed in the tract to keep it open. The Foley should be replaced with a G-tube replacement within 1 week.

## PEG IS CLOGGED

Clogged PEGs do not necessarily have to be replaced. The first step is flushing with warm water or diet soda. An enzymatic declogger such as Viokase (pancrelipase) can also be tried. The last step before replacement would be mechanical cleaning with an endoscopy cleaning brush or a biopsy forceps. If the tube appears old or ready to be replaced, the most prudent step would be to replace it with a new tube.

## PEG TRACT IS INFECTED

The presence of warmth, tenderness, fluctuance, or purulent drainage indicates a possible G-tube tract infection. Tract infections are similar to other skin infections such as cellulitis. Treatment with an oral first-generation cephalosporin for 7 days should cover most skin flora involved in these infections. The tube almost never has to be removed for a tract infection. In the rare instance of a severe infection, intravenous antibiotics or an incision and débridement may be needed.

## PEG IS LEAKING

Leakage of gastric contents or feeding can often be fixed by tightening a loose external bumper. One should resist the urge to replace a leaking tube with a larger tube as this may result in progressive dilation of the tract and more leakage. Occasionally, a long-term tract will not close after a tube is removed, and suturing may be required.

### TISSUE CAUGHT IN TRACT

Occasionally, granulation tissue will be seen in the G-tube tract and will be caught under the external bumper. The contact between the tube and the tract can be very painful and may bleed. Treatment of the tissue with silver nitrate will usually fix the problem. Be aware that silver nitrate treatment can be painful for the patient and may discolor bare skin (black) on contact.

# Jejunostomy Tubes

Jejunostomy tubes are placed distal to the ligament of Treitz. Most are gastronomy/jejunostomy (GJ) tubes in which the jejunostomy tube is threaded through a gastrostomy tube into the small bowel and can be placed either endoscopically or fluoroscopically. GJ tubes are placed for partial gastric outlet obstruction or persistent aspiration with G-tube feedings, but improved aspiration rates have never been proven. Nasojejunal tubes are also placed endoscopically or fluoroscopically for feeding in acute pancreatitis but can be inadvertently pulled out by the patient. Both GJ and nasojejunal tubes often migrate back into the stomach. Similar to surgical G-tubes, surgical jejunostomy tubes are usually placed during other surgical procedures.

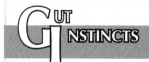

FEEDING TUBES

1. Dedicated NG feeding tubes should be used rather than Salem Sump tubes for feeding. A standard (16F, 36 inches) tube can be used unless postpyloric or long-term feeding would require a small-bore (8F, 45 inches) tube.

2. Gastrostomy tubes can be placed either endoscopically or under fluoroscopic guidance. For near obstructing lesions, fluoroscopic guidance is preferred.

3. Feedings can be advanced as rapidly as 4 hours after gastrostomy tube placement with careful checking of residuals.

4. Do not replace a gastrostomy tube at bedside until the tract is mature (more than 4 weeks old).

5. Jejunostomy tubes are often placed for patients who aspirate on gastrostomy feedings, but they are difficult to place and are prone to migrate back into the stomach.

## Key References

1. McClave SA, Neff RL. Care and long-term maintenance of percutaneous endoscopic gastrostomy tubes. *JPEN J Parenter Enteral Nutr.* 2006;30 (1 Suppl):S27-S38.

2. Nicholson FB, Korman MG, Richardson, MA. Percutaneous endoscopic gastrostomy: a review of indications, complications and outcome. *J Gastroenterol Hepatol.* 2000;15(1):21-25.

3. Schraq SP, Sharma R, Jaik NP, et al. Complications related to percutaneous endoscopic gastrostomy (PEG) tubes. A comprehensive clinical review. *J Gastrointestin Liver Dis.* 2007;16(4):407-418.

# NONVARICEAL UPPER GASTROINTESTINAL BLEEDING

Kevin A. Ghassemi, MD and
Dennis M. Jensen, MD

Upper gastrointestinal (UGI) bleeding occurs proximal to the ligament of Treitz. It presents usually as either hematemesis (vomiting of blood or coffee ground-like material) or melena (black, tarry stool). In about 15% to 20% of severe cases, it can manifest as hematochezia (red blood or clots per rectum). The most common cause of UGI bleeding is from an ulcer (40% of cases). Other causes of UGI bleeding are esophageal or gastric varices (16%), esophagitis (13%), UGI tumor (7%), vascular ectasia (6%), Mallory-Weiss tear (4%), Dieulafoy's lesions and watermelon stomach (2% each). This chapter will discuss the evidence-based approach to evaluation and treatment of nonvariceal causes of UGI bleeding.

## Initial Evaluation

A medical history should be the starting point of the evaluation, with questions looking for risk factors and likelihood of specific bleeding sources. These include chronic liver disease (varices, watermelon stomach), aspirin/nonsteroidal anti-inflammatory drug (NSAID) use (ulcers), chronic kidney disease/dialysis dependence (vascular ectasias), retching/vomiting before bleeding onset (Mallory-Weiss tear), and history of abdominal aortic aneurysm (aorto-enteric fistula). Physical examination should focus on vital signs (evidence of tachycardia, hypotension, and orthostasis) and signs of systemic disease, such as

Esrailian E. *Gut Instincts: A Clinician's Handbook of Digestive and Liver Diseases* (pp 59-64).
© 2012 Taylor & Francis Group

evidence of cirrhosis/portal hypertension. A nasogastric (NG) tube can be helpful to localize melena or hematochezia to a UGI source. A lavage that returns bilious fluid makes it unlikely that the bleeding source is from the UGI tract but does not rule it out. A lavage that returns clear fluid is nondiagnostic. Even if bloody or coffee-ground emesis is witnessed, a NG tube can help clear the stomach of excess blood, improving future endoscopic visualization and reducing the aspiration risk.

## Pre-Endoscopic Management

Resuscitation efforts should begin along with the initial evaluation. Large-bore (14- or 16-gauge) intravenous catheters are recommended, with normal saline infused as fast as necessary to maintain hemodynamic stability. Although each situation is different and data regarding thresholds are limited, the general recommendation is to transfuse blood products as needed to keep the hemoglobin above 8 g/dL, the platelet count above 50,000/mm$^3$, and the international normalized ratio (INR) below 2 prior to endoscopy. Clinicians should consider endotracheal intubation in patients with active hematemesis and/or with altered mental or respiratory status to prevent aspiration.

The most common cause of UGI bleeding is a peptic ulcer. Therefore, if an ulcer bleed is suspected, pre-endoscopic acid suppression therapy should be considered, especially if there may be a delay in endoscopy of more than 12 hours. Pre-endoscopic proton pump inhibitors (PPIs) can downstage the lesion severity and the need for endoscopic therapy, but they do not alter clinical outcomes. Pantoprazole is usually given as an 80-mg intravenous bolus followed by an 8-mg per hour continuous infusion, but dosing can vary depending on the drug used in a given institution.

## Endoscopy

Endoscopy can identify the site of bleeding and provide therapeutic hemostasis in most patients. Patients with evidence of active bleeding (fresh blood on NG lavage or tachycardia/hypotension) should undergo endoscopy as soon as possible after adequate medical resuscitation. An intravenous prokinetic (erythromycin 250 mg or metoclopramide 10 mg) should be considered to help move blood out of the stomach and improve endoscopic visualization.

Ulcers can be classified based on stigmata of recent hemorrhage (SRH; Figure 9-1). High-risk stigmata are arterial spurting, nonbleeding visible vessel (NBVV), and adherent clot (does not dislodge with aggressive washing). Low-risk stigmata are a flat pigmented spot and

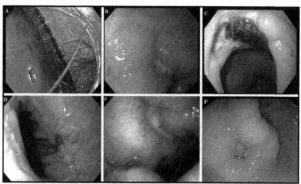

**Figure 9-1.** Stigmata of ulcer hemorrhage. (A) Arterial spurting bleed. (B) Nonbleeding visible vessel. (C) Adherent clot. (D) Oozing without high-risk stigmata. (E) Flat pigmented spot. (F) Clean base.

clean base. Ulcers with oozing blood and no other SRH are considered intermediate-risk. This classification can guide how or whether to treat these lesions endoscopically (Figure 9-2). High-risk ulcers have more than a 33% chance of rebleeding and should undergo combination therapy with 1:20,000 epinephrine (injected submucosally around the SRH) and either thermal coagulation or mechanical compression (hemoclips). Intermediate-risk ulcers have a 10% to 30% risk for rebleeding and should be treated with hemoclipping or thermal coagulation. Combination therapy has been repeatedly shown to be superior to monotherapy. Ulcers with low-risk stigmata are much less likely to rebleed and do not require endoscopic treatment.

Endoscopic treatment can be performed on other UGI bleeding sources in the appropriate setting. Esophagitis and most Mallory-Weiss tears will heal with medical therapy or even spontaneously. However, severe Mallory-Weiss tears can have similar high-risk stigmata on endoscopy as ulcers and should undergo endoscopic treatment with injection and hemoclipping. Dieulafoy's lesions should also be treated with combination endoscopic therapy. Vascular ectasias, including gastric antral vascular ectasias (GAVE; also described as "watermelon stomach"), can be treated endoscopically either with thermal probe or argon plasma coagulation.

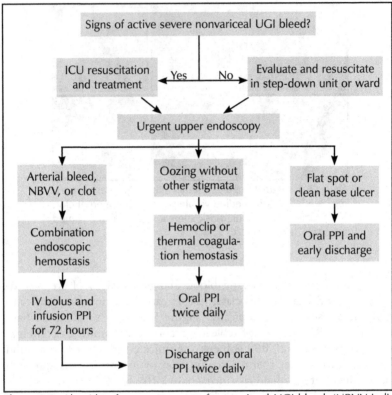

**Figure 9-2.** Algorithm for management of nonvariceal UGI bleed. (NBVV indicates nonbleeding visible vessel; PPI, proton pump inhibitor.)

# Postendoscopic Management and Follow-Up

The SRH can also guide medical therapy after successful endoscopy has been performed. Patients with high-risk stigmata should receive a 72-hour continuous PPI infusion (as described above) after endoscopic hemostasis and should be subsequently converted to oral PPI therapy. Low- and intermediate-risk stigmata patients can be started on oral PPIs with observation or discharge as dictated by the clinical setting. PPIs can be used to accelerate healing of Mallory-Weiss tears and should be used in patients with erosive esophagitis.

Patients with UGI bleeds due to peptic ulcers should be checked for *Helicobacter pylori* infection and treated appropriately to reduce the risk of recurrent peptic ulcers. Patients with gastric ulcers should be considered for follow-up endoscopy after approximately 6 to 8 weeks of

PPI therapy to assess for healing and any underlying gastric malignancy. Esophagitis patients should have a repeat endoscopy after 8 weeks of PPI treatment to assess for underlying Barrett's esophagus. Several sessions of endoscopic coagulation, 4 to 8 weeks apart, may be needed to eradicate GAVE. In general, Mallory-Weiss tears, Dieulafoy's lesions, and isolated vascular ectasias do not require follow-up unless there is clinically significant recurrent bleeding.

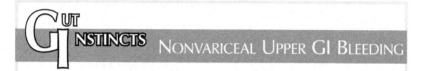

1. In patients with upper gastrointestinal bleeding, assessment of vital signs and nasogastric lavage can help determine bleeding severity and the urgency for performing endoscopy.

2. Pre-endoscopic PPI therapy can downstage lesion severity and reduce the need for endoscopic therapy, but it should not delay the endoscopy.

3. High- and intermediate-risk ulcers should undergo endoscopic treatment and have high-dose PPIs afterward for 72 hours, whereas patients with low-risk ulcers can be treated with oral PPIs and be considered for early discharge.

4. Combination endoscopic therapy has been repeatedly shown to be superior to monotherapy.

5. Watermelon stomach and vascular ectasias can be treated with either thermal probe or argon plasma coagulation.

## Key References

1. Barkun AN, Bardou M, Kuipers EJ, et al. International consensus recommendations on the management of patients with nonvariceal upper gastrointestinal bleeding. *Ann Intern Med.* 2010;152(2):101-113.

2. Gralnek IM, Barkun AN, Bardou M. Management of acute bleeding from a peptic ulcer. *N Engl J Med.* 2008;359(9):928-937.

# CHAPTER 10

# ACID-PEPTIC DISORDERS

Thomas O. G. Kovacs, MD

Peptic ulcer disease (PUD) occurs commonly and is an important cause of morbidity and health care costs. Although the incidence of PUD has decreased over the past decade (yearly incidence of 5 cases per 1000 people), the rates of hospitalization and deaths from ulcer complications have been relatively stable over that same time. A peptic ulcer is a defect in the gastric or duodenal wall that extends through the muscularis mucosa (the deepest limit of the mucosa) into the submucosa or muscularis propria.

## Pathogenesis

The gastric lumen pH is about 1, while the gastric mucosal barrier maintains a pH of approximately 7 at the mucosal surface. Tissue injury is avoided through a balance between aggressive factors, such as *Helicobacter pylori* (Hp) infection and acid and pepsin secretion, and defensive factors, such as mucosal blood flow and bicarbonate and mucus secretion. Altering this balance leads to ulcer formation. Most ulcers develop secondary to Hp infection, increased secretion, and nonsteroidal anti-inflammatory drug (NSAID) use.

### HELICOBACTER PYLORI

Hp is a gram-negative bacterium found on the luminal surface of the gastric epithelium that induces chronic mucosal inflammation. The

Esrailian E. *Gut Instincts: A Clinician's Handbook of Digestive and Liver Diseases* (pp 65-70).
© 2012 Taylor & Francis Group

infection usually occurs in the first few years of life and persists unless treated. At least 50% of the world's population is infected with Hp. Hp infection is an important co-factor in the development of duodenal or gastric ulcers, occurring in 1% to 10% of infected patients. About 90% of patients with duodenal ulcer and 60% to 70% of those with gastric ulcer are Hp positive. Hp eradication leads to ulcer healing and a substantially reduced recurrence rate. The exact mechanism(s) underlying Hp's ulcerogenesis are not well understood. Epithelial surface changes, local pH alteration, toxin production, gastrin stimulation, as well as other host factors have all been implicated.

Hp has also been identified as a co-factor in gastric cancer (in 0.1% to 1%) and gastric mucosa-associated lymphoid-tissue (MALT) lymphoma (in <0.01%). Despite these associations, most Hp-infected patients will not have any clinically important conditions.

## ACID SECRETION

"No acid, no ulcer" may still be true in the Hp era, because peptic ulcer virtually never occurs in the absence of acid and heals with reduction of acid secretion. Acid over-production is seen in only 30% to 50% of duodenal ulcer patients, and other factors are also important in the development of peptic ulcers. Zollinger-Ellison syndrome, due to a gastrin-secreting pancreatic or duodenal non-beta islet cell tumor, results in gastric acid hypersecretion. It is the best example of ulcer disease associated with profound acid overproduction.

## NONSTEROIDAL ANTI-INFLAMMATORY DRUG USE

NSAID use is closely associated with an increased risk of developing ulcers. Studies show that up to 75% of patients have endoscopic injury of the UGI tract after even brief courses of NSAIDs, and 50% to 60% of hospitalized UGI bleeding patients admit to NSAID ingestion in the week prior to their hemorrhage. NSAID-induced ulcers develop secondary to the systemic inhibition of prostaglandin production, which is involved in mucosal repair and circulation.

# Presentation

Dyspepsia, or upper abdominal discomfort, is the most frequent symptom in PUD patients. It is often described as gnawing or a hunger pain, and it tends to occur when the stomach is empty or overnight. Food and antacids usually improve symptoms, although in some patients eating exacerbates the discomfort. Hematemesis, vomiting, melena, pain radiating into the back, and severe abdominal pain with peritoneal signs may indicate the development of a complication of ulcer disease such as GI hemorrhage, gastric outlet obstruction, penetration (erosion of ulcer through the serosa into adjacent tissues such as the pancreas), or perforation.

## Diagnosis

Although most cases of dyspepsia have no organic cause, PUD is noted in 5% to 15% of dyspeptic patients. Recent guidelines recommend upper endoscopy in patients older than age 50 with new-onset dyspepsia and in patients of any age with alarm features, such as unintended weight loss, overt GI hemorrhage, vomiting, a palpable mass or lymphadenopathy, or a family history of UGI malignancy. In dyspeptic patients younger than age 50 years without alarm features, Hp infection should be evaluated and treated if testing is positive. If patients are on NSAIDs, the medication should be stopped if possible. Patients who are Hp negative should have either empiric acid suppression for 4 to 8 weeks or an upper endoscopy. In uncomplicated PUD, the role of endoscopy is to confirm the diagnosis and exclude malignancy.

## Testing for *Helicobacter pylori*

Patients with confirmed duodenal or gastric ulcer, gastric MALT lymphoma, and resection of early gastric cancer, and young patients with uncomplicated dyspepsia should be tested. Evaluation of Hp infection (Table 10-1) may be categorized into nonendoscopic and endoscopic tests. The nonendoscopic tests include serologic, fecal antigen, and urea-breath tests. These tests are accurate with good sensitivity and specificity, but with certain limitations. Serologic testing is of limited value in confirming eradication of infection. The fecal antigen and urea breath tests require discontinuing antimicrobial agents for 4 weeks and proton pump inhibitors (PPIs) for 2 weeks prior to testing. These medications may decrease the tests' sensitivity by suppressing the infection. Endoscopic tests include urease-based biopsy tests, histologic examination, and culture. Testing should also be performed to confirm Hp eradication in patients who have had ulcer, gastric MALT lymphoma, resected gastric cancer, and in those patients whose symptoms persist after Hp eradication therapy for dyspepsia.

## Treatment

The goals of therapy include ulcer healing, symptom relief, and prevention of recurrences and complications. For PUD patients who test positive for Hp, several drug regimens are effective. Most involve a PPI or a bismuth compound (or both) and 2 antibiotics.

| TABLE 10-1 | TESTS USED TO DETECT *HELICOBACTER PYLORI* INFECTION | |
|---|---|---|
| **Test** | **Advantages** | **Disadvantages** |
| *Nonendoscopic* | | |
| Serologic | Cheap, widely available | Positive test may indicate prior not current infection; not useful to confirm eradication. |
| Urea breath | Highly accurate; useful pre- and post-Rx | PPIs, B, and antibiotics may cause false-negative results |
| Fecal antigen | Highly accurate; useful pre- and post-Rx | PPIs, B, and antibiotics may cause false-negative results |
| *Endoscopic* | | |
| Urea-based biopsy | Accurate and rapid | PPIs, B, and antibiotics may cause false- negative results |
| Histology | Very accurate | Requires specialized training |
| Culture | High specificity; Allows test of antibiotic sensitivity | Variable sensitivity; Needs specialized staff and facilities |
| PPI indicates proton pump inhibitor; B, bismuth preparation; Rx, therapy | | |

One of the most frequently used regimens is a PPI plus amoxicillin and clarithromycin, each taken twice daily, for 10 to 14 days (7 days in Europe). Metronidazole may replace amoxicillin in penicillin allergy patients. For patients who fail initial therapy, bismuth-based quadruple with a PPI twice daily, bismuth, and tetracycline and metronidazole (each 4 times a day for 10 to 14 days) has been successful in 57% to 95% of cases.

Antisecretory therapy with a PPI is also indicated for 4 to 6 weeks, except in patients with a smaller (<1 cm) uncomplicated ulcer in whom Hp eradication therapy usually produces healing. Continued antisecretory treatment with a PPI is indicated in patients with larger ulcers (>1 cm), complicated ulcers, and until Hp eradication is confirmed. After Hp eradication and stopping NSAIDs, duodenal ulcer healing occurs in more than 90% of duodenal ulcer patients.

PUD patients on NSAIDs should be treated with a PPI, and NSAIDs should be stopped whenever possible. If NSAID use is unavoidable, the lowest dose should be used, and PPI co-therapy should continue as long as NSAIDs are taken.

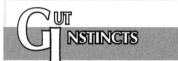

ACID-PEPTIC DISORDERS

1. Hp infection, nonsteroidal anti-inflammatory drug use, and acid overproduction are important for ulcer development.
2. Testing for the presence of Hp should be performed in all patients with PUD.
3. Hp is associated with PUD, gastric cancer, and gastric mucosa-associated lymphoid tissue.
4. The first-line treatment for Hp consists of a PPI and 2 antibiotics (eg, PPI, clarithromycin, amoxicillin) twice daily for 10 to 14 days.
5. In older patients (>55 years of age), those with new-onset dyspepsia, and/or in the setting of alarm features such as weight loss, dysphagia, vomiting, gastrointestinal bleeding, or a family history of an upper gastrointestinal malignancy, an upper endoscopy is recommended.

## Key References

1. McColl KEL. *Helicobacter pylori* infection. *N Engl J Med.* 2010;362(17): 1597-1604.
2. ASGE Standards of Practice Committee. The role of endoscopy in the management of patients with peptic ulcer disease. *Gastrointestinal Endoscopy.* 2011;71(4):663-668.

# CHAPTER 11

# FUNCTIONAL DYSPEPSIA

Richard J. Saad, MD, MS and
William D. Chey, MD, AGAF, FACG, FACP

*Dyspepsia* is a term used to describe a constellation of symptoms believed to arise from the gastroduodenal region of the gastrointestinal (GI) tract. Symptoms include postprandial fullness and epigastric pain or burning. Accompanying symptoms include nausea, vomiting, bloating, belching, and weight loss. After excluding structural and organic etiologies, this symptom complex is termed *functional dyspepsia* (FD). Dyspepsia is highly prevalent with the majority of cases attributed to FD. Specific symptoms, frequency, and severity often vary over time. FD frequently overlaps with other functional bowel disorders such as nonerosive reflux disease and irritable bowel syndrome (IBS).

## Differential Diagnosis

Common causes of dyspepsia include gastroesophageal reflux disease (GERD) and peptic ulcer disease (PUD). Malignancies are rare causes of dyspeptic symptoms, occurring in fewer than 1% of cases in the United States. Although celiac disease and carbohydrate maldigestion/malabsorption (lactose, fructose, sorbitol, and mannitol) are most commonly associated with lower GI symptoms such as bloating, flatulence, and diarrhea, they can occasionally present with dyspeptic symptoms. Gastroparesis is defined by the presence of delayed gastric emptying. The symptoms of gastroparesis and FD are difficult, if not impossible, to distinguish. In fact, 30% to 40% of patients diagnosed with FD have

Esrailian E. *Gut Instincts: A Clinician's Handbook of Digestive and Liver Diseases* (pp 71-76).
© 2012 Taylor & Francis Group

delayed gastric emptying by scintigraphy. Rare upper GI tract inflammatory and infiltrative conditions presenting with dyspepsia include Crohn's disease, pancreatitis, sarcoidosis, and amyloidosis. Nonsteroidal anti-inflammatory drugs (NSAIDs) and aspirin are medications most commonly associated with the development of dyspeptic symptoms. Any medication can cause dyspepsia if a temporal relationship exists between therapy and symptoms. Systemic diseases including diabetes mellitus, thyroid disease, parathyroid disorders, and connective tissue disorders can be associated with dyspeptic symptoms. Other rare causes of dyspepsia include intestinal ischemia, liver or pancreatic malignancy, and hyperkalemia. Pregnancy should always be considered in a woman presenting with dyspepsia, particularly when nausea predominates.

## Diagnostic Approach

Patients with FD are distinguished from those with uninvestigated dyspepsia only after excluding structural disease, such as with endoscopy or imaging. Endoscopy is preferred given its diagnostic accuracy and ability to obtain mucosal biopsies. Endoscopy should be performed in patients with uninvestigated dyspepsia who are older than 50 years or have alarm features at any age (melena, weight loss, anorexia, early satiety, persistent vomiting, dysphagia, odynophagia, family history of upper GI malignancy, personal history of PUD or malignancy, prior gastric surgery, or anemia). It is also appropriate to perform endoscopy for persistent dyspepsia despite the "test and treat" strategy for *Helicobacter pylori* and/or a 4-week or longer trial of proton pump inhibitor (PPI) therapy.

Testing beyond endoscopy is generally of low yield and should be considered depending on the specific patient circumstances.

## Pathophysiology

The pathogenesis of FD remains poorly defined. Purported mechanisms include abnormal upper GI motor and reflex functions, visceral hypersensitivity, altered brain-gut interactions, disrupted gut-immune interactions, psychological factors, and genetic factors. Unfortunately, identifiable physiological abnormalities do not closely correlate with the specific symptoms. Postprandial fullness, nausea, and vomiting are more common in FD patients with delayed gastric emptying; however, many FD patients with normal gastric emptying will have the same symptoms. This fact underscores a heterogeneous pathophysiology.

# Management Strategies

Treatment is largely predicated on relieving primary symptoms. Because no single therapy is universally effective in patients with FD, many patients require more than one empiric treatment trial before achieving symptom improvement. Options include dietary modifications, over-the-counter (OTC) and prescription medications, psychological treatments, and complementary and alternative medicine (CAM) therapies (Table 11-1).

## DIETARY AND LIFESTYLE MEASURES

The use of dietary therapy stems from the observation that symptoms are frequently associated with or exacerbated by food. Many of the recommendations for GERD also apply to patients with FD. Ingesting smaller, more frequent meals and avoiding late evening meals can be of benefit. Fatty foods have effects on gastric emptying and sensation and are commonly associated with symptoms and, thus, should be avoided. With documented delays in gastric emptying, a trial with a low-residue diet may help. It may be helpful for the patient to maintain a food diary for a period of 2 weeks in the hopes of identifying culprit behaviors or foods. Implicated behaviors or foods can then be reduced or eliminated.

## PHARMACOLOGIC THERAPY

Successful *H. pylori* eradication is effective in a small subset of patients. A 10- to 14-day course of therapy is recommended. Shorter durations have demonstrated efficacy outside of the United States. Antisecretory drugs including PPIs and histamine-2-receptor antagonists (H$_2$RAs) provide reasonably safe and effective treatment options. PPIs are the best studied and most effective agents of the antisecretory drug class. PPIs are most effective in FD patients who report epigastric pain or who report concurrent heartburn and are least effective in those with motility-related symptoms such as nausea and bloating. Antacids, bismuth-based products, and sucralfate appear no more effective than placebo in clinical trials.

Prokinetics should be reserved for FD cases with delayed gastric emptying. The term *prokinetic* refers to drugs with varied effects of gastric function and sensation. Generally, prokinetics accelerate gastric emptying. The dopaminergic antagonist metoclopramide possesses prokinetic and antiemetic properties, making it attractive for use in FD. Unfortunately, metoclopramide crosses the blood-brain barrier and is associated with the development of central nervous system side effects

| TABLE 11-1 | PHARMACOLOGIC TREATMENTS FOR FUNCTIONAL DYSPEPSIA |
|---|---|
| **Drug Class** | **Dosing Instructions** |
| *Proton Pump Inhibitors* | |
| Dexlansoprazole Esomeprazole Lansoprazole Omeprazole Pantoprazole Rabeprazole | 4-week trial using standard dose Consider additional 4-week trial at higher dose given once or twice daily |
| *Histamine Receptor Antagonists* | |
| Ranitidine Famotidine Cimetidine | 2- to 4-week trial at over-the-counter (OTC) dose Consider another 2 to 4 weeks at double the recommended OTC dose |
| *Prokinetics* | |
| Metoclopramide | Initial dose of 5 to 10 mg, 4 times daily Maximum dose of 20 mg, 4 times daily |
| *Tricyclic Antidepressants* | |
| Amitriptyline Desipramine Nortriptyline | Initial dose of 10 mg every night at bedtime 1 to 2 weeks at starting dose Increase by 10 mg aliquots Maximum dose of 50 mg/day |
| *Selective Serotonin Reuptake Inhibitors* | |
| Citalopram Escitalopram Fluoxetine Paroxetine Sertraline | 4-week trial using standard initial dose |
| *Serotonin Norepinephrine Reuptake Inhibitors* | |
| Duloextine Venlafaxine | 4-week trial using standard initial dose |

including anxiety, dysphoria, insomnia, and dystonia in up to 20% of patients. Furthermore, metoclopramide can rarely cause the irreversible side effect of tardive dyskinesia. Domperidone is a peripherally acting dopaminergic antagonist offering the benefits of metoclopramide without the same side effects. Domperidone is available in most countries around the world but is not available in the United States. Both of these drugs can increase prolactin levels and rarely have been associated with cardiac arrhythmias. The motilin agonist erythromycin possesses potent gastrokinetic properties, but negatively affects gastric accommodation and is subject to the development of tolerance with extended use.

Drugs with more central than peripheral effects, including antidepressants and anxiolytics, may be considered. Antidepressants include tricyclic agents (TCAs), selective serotonin reuptake inhibitors (SSRIs), or serotonin norepinephrine reuptake inhibitors (SNRIs). There is more evidence supporting the use of antidepressants in patients with IBS than FD. In general, TCAs are most effective for treating pain while SSRIs and SNRIs tend to offer greater benefits to patients with anxiety or significant life stress. Side effects of TCAs include dry mouth and eyes, constipation, drowsiness, and weight gain, which may limit their use. Therefore, starting at the lowest available dose and gradually titrating up over a period of weeks provides the greatest likelihood of success.

## PSYCHOLOGICAL THERAPY

Psychological therapy may be considered if FD symptoms are linked to anxiety or stress or for those with a history of abuse or comorbid psychological conditions. Possible modalities include psychodrama, cognitive behavioral therapy, relaxation therapy, guided imagery, and hypnotherapy. Out-of-pocket expenses, the stigma attached to such therapies, and availability of trained therapists often limit their practical utility.

## COMPLEMENTARY AND ALTERNATIVE MEDICINE

Use of herbal products has grown in popularity. The best-studied agents include STW 5 (Iberogast, Steigarwald, Darmstadt, Germany), peppermint, and caraway with some evidence also suggesting a benefit with capsaicin and artichoke leaf extract. Herbal remedies are currently regulated as food additives and, as such, are not subject to the quality standards that apply to pharmaceuticals. Furthermore, safety data and drug interactions are often unknown.

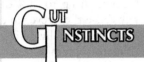

**FUNCTIONAL DYSPEPSIA**

1. Organic/structural disease must be excluded before the diagnosis of functional dyspepsia can be made.
2. Functional dyspepsia may overlap with other functional bowel disorders, such as irritable bowel syndrome and nonerosive reflux disease.
3. Upper endoscopy is the diagnostic study of choice for the evaluation of dyspepsia.
4. Patients age 50 and older with dyspeptic symptoms, and those with alarm features at any age, should be further evaluated with an upper endoscopy.
5. Due to the heterogeneous nature of functional dyspepsia, no universally effective treatment exists.

## Key References

1. Talley NJ, Vakil NB, Moayyedi P. American Gastroenterological Association technical review on the evaluation of dyspepsia. *Gastroenterology.* 2005;129(5): 1756-1780.
2. Saad RJ, Chey WD. Review article: current and emerging therapies for functional dyspepsia. *Aliment Pharmacol Ther.* 2006;24(3):475-492.
3. Tack J, Talley NJ, Camilleri M, et al. Functional gastroduodenal disorders. *Gastroenterology. 2006;*130(5):1466-1479.

# CHAPTER 12

# PANCREATIC DISEASES

James Farrell, MD

## Acute Pancreatitis

### DIAGNOSIS

The diagnosis of acute pancreatitis is based on a combination of both clinical (severe epigastric pain radiating to the back, relieved by sitting forward) and laboratory tests (elevated amylase and lipase [more specific] blood levels). The absolute value of the amylase and lipase blood level is not predictive of the severity or natural history of an attack of acute pancreatitis. Initial abdominal magnetic resonance imaging (MRI) or computed tomography (CT) scan imaging is not necessary unless there is some doubt about the initial diagnosis. An abdominal ultrasound is more useful to identify gallstones as a possible etiology. While the most likely cause for acute pancreatitis is gallstones and alcohol, other common causes include medications, elevated triglycerides, hypercalcemia, abdominal trauma, postendoscopic retrograde cholangiopancreatography (ERCP) pancreatitis, and pancreas divisum. Inherited cause of pancreatitis should be considered if there is a strong family history of pancreatitis or an onset before 35 years of age. In a patient older than 40, the first attack of pancreatitis should raise the suspicion of an underlying pancreatic cyst or mass.

Esrailian E. *Gut Instincts: A Clinician's Handbook of Digestive and Liver Diseases* (pp 77-84).
© 2012 Taylor & Francis Group

## MANAGEMENT

Most patients with an attack of acute pancreatitis settle down within 5 to 7 days with appropriate bowel rest, intravenous fluids, correction of electrolyte and metabolic abnormalities, and analgesia. A small group may have a prolonged course with systemic disturbances (10% to 15%), often requiring intensive care unit (ICU) management, and rarely resulting in death (<3%). This subgroup can be identified earlier at the time of presentation or after 48 to 72 hours of hospitalization using a combination of clinical, laboratory, and radiologic risk factors: elevated hematocrit, elevated white blood cell count, organ failure (renal or lung), age (>75 years), comorbid illness, and alcoholic pancreatitis. The best validated scoring system to predict severity of acute pancreatitis is the Acute Physiology and Chronic Health Evaluation (APACHE) II scoring system (using a cutoff of 8). In patients with a predicted severe course, actual organ failure, or a suspicion of infection, a contrast CT scan may be indicated to assess for degree of pancreatic necrosis after 72 hours.

For most patients with mild acute pancreatitis, soft diet can be started after resolution of pain. For patients with severe pancreatitis, enteral nutrition (if possible) is preferred to parenteral nutrition. The role of prophylactic antibiotic for the management of pancreatic necrosis remains controversial. However, surgery should be considered in patients with infected pancreatic necrosis. For presumed biliary pancreatitis, urgent ERCP (defined as within 72 hours) is indicated for worsening biliary obstruction, ascending cholangitis, and severe pancreatitis. Cholecystectomy should be performed subsequently in all patients with gallstone pancreatitis. While most patients with acute pancreatitis will improve within 24 to 48 hours, prolonged symptoms should raise concerns about the development of pancreatic fluid collections.

# Chronic Pancreatitis

## DIAGNOSIS

Chronic pancreatitis is defined histologically as irreversible pancreatic gland destruction with fibrosis, which can result in impaired exocrine and endocrine dysfunction. However, up to 90% of the pancreas gland needs to be affected before endocrine or exocrine dysfunction is clinically apparent. Making the diagnosis of chronic pancreatitis clinically can be difficult in the absence of clinical evidence of fat malabsorption or glucose intolerance, or the classic radiologic findings of pancreatic calcification, intraductal pancreatic stones, or a dilated pancreatic duct.

Often, endoscopic ultrasound (EUS) examination is preferred to ERCP to make the diagnosis of early chronic pancreatitis, although this can be overly sensitive. Pancreatic function testing is not widely available. While the most common cause of chronic pancreatitis remains alcohol, other important causes include hereditary pancreatitis (cystic fibrosis transmembrane conductance regulator [CFTRgene], serine proteinase inhibitor Kazal Type 1 [SPINK-1] gene, protease, serine, 1 [trypsin 1] [PRSS-1] gene) and autoimmune pancreatitis (AIP). Identifying a cause is important to lessen the development of repeat attacks and to risk-stratify the patient for cancer risk. Making the diagnosis of AIP (elevated immunoglobulin G4, hyperintense peripancreatic "halo" on CT scan) is important because some of these patients may respond to treatment with steroids.

## MANAGEMENT

Management of chronic pancreatitis is aimed at identifying and treating the complications including pain, exocrine insufficiency, endocrine insufficiency, glucose intolerance (diabetes mellitus), biliary obstruction, splenic vein occlusion, pseudocyst formation, bile duct or duodenal obstruction, and increased cancer risk. The management of pain associated with chronic pancreatitis is primarily medical (analgesia and a trial of pancreatic enzymes), with a limited role for celiac nerve block or endoscopic therapy. Surgical management for pain control (pancreatic resection, lateral pancreaticojejunostomy) may be warranted and appears to be superior to endoscopic therapy long-term. Exocrine insufficiency is typically managed with pancreatic enzymes and restriction of fat intake titrated to correct fat malabsorption, resolve steatorrhea, and maintain weight. Concomitant gastric acid inhibition is necessary to avoid acid inactivation of uncoated pancreatic enzymes. Long-term biliary obstruction is best managed through surgical biliary diversion or occasionally by endoscopic stenting to avoid the development of secondary biliary cirrhosis. The risk of cancer associated with chronic pancreatitis varies with the underlying etiology, with patients with hereditary pancreatitis having the highest risk. While routine screening for pancreatic cancer in patients with chronic pancreatitis is not recommended, the development of an acute change in a previously stable patient with chronic pancreatitis (weight loss, biliary obstruction, worsening pain, elevated carbohydrate antigen 19-9) should prompt a search for an underlying malignancy.

# Pancreatic Masses

Although there is a broad differential diagnosis for a pancreatic mass, for patients over the age of 40, the diagnosis is pancreatic adenocarcinoma until proven otherwise. Other diagnoses include pancreatic endocrine tumors (younger patients, atypical findings on imaging, lack of biliary or pancreatic duct obstruction), associated familial syndrome (multiple endocrine neoplasia Type 1), metastases (breast cancer, renal cancer), or focal chronic pancreatitis (such as in autoimmune pancreatitis). Jaundice, abdominal pain, and weight loss are common presenting symptoms of patients with pancreatic masses. Pancreatic head masses tend to present earlier due to biliary obstruction than those in the pancreatic body or tail.

Evaluation of a presumed pancreatic adenocarcinoma begins with a good quality CT or MRI scan looking for evidence of locally advanced disease (involving the portal vein, superior mesenteric vein, or superior mesenteric artery) or metastatic disease. If there is evidence of locally advanced disease or metastases, then a tissue diagnosis (either by CT-guided biopsy or EUS-guided biopsy) of the primary or metastatic lesion followed by chemotherapy is indicated. Otherwise, evaluation for surgical resection is warranted. Preoperative biliary stent placement for jaundice is indicated for pruritus, cholangitis, or a prolonged delay prior to surgical resection. Preoperative tissue diagnosis may be warranted for a pancreatic mass in which the diagnosis is unclear, although a negative biopsy does not exclude the possibility of an underlying cancer. While EUS-guided biopsy of the head of the pancreas transduodenally is considered safe, transgastric biopsy of potentially resectable pancreatic body and tail masses carries the risk of tumor seeding.

# Pancreatic Cysts

Pancreatic cysts are increasingly diagnosed due to the widespread prevalence of radiologic imaging for unrelated conditions. Although there are many uncommon types of pancreatic cysts (solid pseudopapillary neoplasms, cystic lymphangioma), pancreatic cysts can be classified broadly as either malignant/premalignant (intraductal papillary mucinous neoplasm [IPMN], mucinous cystic neoplasm [MCN], or malignant degeneration of a solid tumor [adenocarcinoma, endocrine]) or low/no malignant potential (pancreatic pseudocyst or serous cystadenoma). For IPMNs arising predominantly from the main pancreatic duct (main duct IPMN), there is a very high risk of coincident cancer.

For IPMN arising from the branches of the pancreatic duct (branch duct IPMN), the risk of having or developing cancer is much lower. Mucinous cystic neoplasms typically occur in the pancreatic body and tail in middle-aged women and carry a high risk of malignancy. Pancreatic pseudocysts typically arise in the setting of acute pancreatitis but often no history of pancreatitis is available at the time of presentation. Serous cystadenomas are predominantly microcystic lesions often with a central stellate scar on imaging. They are often asymptomatic but may present abdominal discomfort or biliary obstruction.

The presumptive diagnosis of pancreatic cysts is made based on a combination of clinical (previous history of pancreatitis), radiologic, endoscopic (gaping "fish mouth ampulla" of IPMN), and endosonographic findings, in addition to cyst fluid analysis. Typically, elevated pancreatic cyst fluid carcinoembryonic antigen (CEA) more than 192 mg/mL favors a mucinous lesion such as an IPMN or an MCN (with an 80% accuracy), but the absolute cyst fluid CEA level does not correlate with the presence of malignancy. A very low CEA (<5 ng/mL) is seen in patients with serous cystadenoma.

All presumed main duct IPMN and MCNs should be considered for surgical resection based on the extent of pancreas involvement. For branch duct IPMNs, surgical resection should be considered for patients with symptoms referable to their pancreatic cyst, for pancreatic cyst size larger than 3 cm, and for pancreatic cyst size smaller than 3 cm when there is associated evidence of a focal mass or a dilated pancreatic duct (Table 12-1). Otherwise, yearly surveillance with a combination of MRI or CT is indicated for these presumed branch duct IPMN. For presumed serous cystadenomas, surgical resection is indicated for symptomatic cysts (abdominal pain or biliary obstruction). Symptomatic pancreatic pseudocysts can be drained endoscopically, percutaneously, or surgically.

| TABLE 12-1 | GUIDELINES FOR MANAGEMENT OF PRESUMED BRANCH DUCT INTRADUCTAL PAPILLARY MUCINOUS NEOPLASM |
| --- | --- |

**Resection Is Indicated if One or More Is Present:**
- Symptoms attributable to the cyst
- Dilatation of the main pancreatic duct more than 6 mm
- Cyst size larger than 30 mm
- Presence of intramural nodules
- Cyst fluid cytology suspicious or positive for malignancy

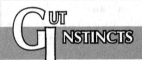

**PANCREATIC DISEASES**

1. For patients with severe pancreatitis, enteral nutrition (if possible) is preferred to parenteral nutrition.
2. Although not always present, chronic pancreatitis has classic findings: fat malabsorption, glucose intolerance, pancreatic calcifications on imaging, intraductal pancreatic stones, and a dilated pancreatic duct.
3. For patients older than age 40, the diagnosis of a pancreatic mass is adenocarcinoma until proven otherwise.
4. Pancreatic head masses tend to present earlier due to biliary obstruction than those in the pancreatic body or tail.
5. For IPMN arising predominantly from the main pancreatic duct (main duct IPMN), there is a very high risk of coincident cancer. The risk in IPMN arising from the branches of the pancreatic duct (branch duct IPMN) is much lower.

# Key References

1. Frossard JL, Steer ML, Pastor CM. Acute pancreatitis. *Lancet*. 2008;371(9607): 143-152.

2. Etemad B, Whitcomb DC. Chronic pancreatitis: diagnosis, classification, and new genetic developments. *Gastroenterology*. 2001;120(3):682-707.

3. Hidalgo M. Pancreatic cancer. *N Engl J Med*. 2010;362(17):1605-1617.

4. Brugge WR, Lauwers GY, Sahani D, Fernandez-del Castillo C, Warshaw AL. Pancreatic cystic neoplasms. *N Engl J Med*. 2004;351(12):1218-1226.

# CHAPTER 13

# BILIARY DISEASES

Yasser M. Bhat, MD and
Inder M. Singh, MD

This chapter focuses on an overview of the diagnosis and management of commonly encountered biliary diseases.

## Acute Cholecystitis

Acute inflammation of the gallbladder resulting in pain, fevers, and leukocytosis.

### PRESENTATION

The typical presentation is fevers, severe right upper quadrant pain, and possibly nausea and vomiting. The pain will often last hours and may radiate to the back or right shoulder. Classically, the pain will occur with intake of a large fatty meal. Of note, the presentation of acute cholecystitis is different from biliary colic, which is often transient and should not be accompanied by fevers. The differential for this presentation is broad and includes acute hepatitis, pancreatitis, and cholangitis.

### PHYSICAL EXAMINATION

The patient may be febrile and tachycardic. The abdominal examination might reveal severe right upper quadrant pain with rebound and guarding. The classical physical finding associated with acute cholecystitis is the presence of deep pain with inspiration occurring

Esrailian E. *Gut Instincts: A Clinician's Handbook of Digestive and Liver Diseases* (pp 85-94).
© 2012 Taylor & Francis Group

while the examiner has fingers pressed in gallbladder fossa below the costal margin (Murphy's sign). This test is sensitive but not specific for this entity.

## LAB STUDIES

Leukocytosis with mild elevation in total bilirubin is seen often. If marked elevation in bilirubin is noted, one must have a low index of suspicion for choledocholithiasis and cholangitis. It is not uncommon for the patient to have mildly elevated transaminases, but these should be no more than 2 to 8 times the upper limit of normal. If higher, an acute hepatitis should be considered.

## IMAGING CHARACTERISTICS

First-line imaging is with abdominal ultrasound. Transabdominal ultrasound may reveal the classic findings of gallstones, gallbladder wall thickening, pericholecystic fluid, and a sonographic Murphy's sign. The combination of these findings in the appropriate clinical setting is highly sensitive and specific for acute cholecystitis. A hepatobiliary (HIDA) scan can be used to help support diagnosis of cholecystitis, especially in cases in which acute cholecystitis is still suspected, but clinical presentation or imaging studies are not typical. Clinicians should not rely on this study when the patient's total bilirubin is greater than 5 because this may lead to a false-positive result.

## MANAGEMENT

All patients diagnosed with acute cholecystitis should be admitted for further care including intravenous hydration and broad-spectrum antibiotics. The patient should remain on nothing by mouth order, and surgical consultation should be obtained. The timing of surgery will depend on the patient's clinical response. If marked response is noted, the patient may undergo elective cholecystectomy when inflammation has settled. If the patient is noted to clinically deteriorate, he or she should be considered for definitive surgical management of possible gangrenous cholecystitis. For a patient who is high risk for surgical intervention, percutaneous drainage (percutaneous cholecystostomy) should be considered.

## PEARLS/PITFALLS

- Do not be fooled by the absence of gallstones. Approximately 10% to 20% of severe acute cases are from acalculous cholecystitis, especially in the sick and elderly.

- Elderly patients can often present atypically.
- Patients with diabetes are more prone to develop emphysematous cholecystitis. This requires early surgical management.

# Biliary Colic and Choledocholithiasis

## PRESENTATION

Gallstones are common and are usually not the focus of any particular attention until they cause symptoms or complications. The presence of cholelithiasis increases with age, and symptoms are generally a result of migration of stones out of the gallbladder. Biliary colic will often occur when stones become impacted in the gallbladder neck and cause a transient obstruction and dilation of the gallbladder. In other instances, the stones may actually pass out of the gallbladder and become trapped in the bile duct. Choledocholithiasis can lead to biliary obstruction, cholangitis, and/or pancreatitis and must be treated.

## LAB STUDIES

With uncomplicated biliary colic, no laboratory abnormalities are expected. As stones migrate out of the gallbladder, tests may become abnormal. Patients with cholangitis will have elevated total bilirubin (direct predominant), leukocytosis, mild transaminitis, and an elevated alkaline phosphatase. In gallstone pancreatitis, concurrent elevations of both amylase and lipase may be noted. With simple choledocholithiasis, the tests may be normal, or elevations of transaminases (ie, twice the upper limit of normal) may be seen.

## IMAGING CHARACTERISTICS

The usual first-line study to approach the diagnosis of stone disease is the transabdominal ultrasound. This study is sensitive, noninvasive, inexpensive, and with almost no risk to the patient. The test is useful for detection of stone disease but is limited in its ability to detect sludge, microlithiasis, and common bile duct stones. If choledocholithiasis is suspected, magnetic resonance cholangiopancreatography (MRCP) should be considered. This test is highly sensitive and specific for the diagnosis of choledocholithiasis. In those patients where MRCP is not possible (ie, metal prosthesis), endoscopic ultrasound (EUS) should be the next study. EUS has been shown to have the same, if not higher, sensitivity to MRCP for detection of choledocholithiasis. The prior gold standard for detection of choledocholithiasis had been endoscopic retrograde cholangiopancreatography (ERCP). This test is no longer used

**Figure 13-1.** ERCP revealing distal common bile duct stone.

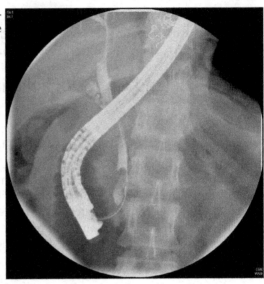

for purely diagnostic purposes given its risk of complications including post-ERCP pancreatitis, infection, and perforation.

## MANAGEMENT

Patients with typical biliary colic and imaging suggestive of cholelithiasis should undergo elective cholecystectomy. Although suboptimal, patients reluctant to undergo cholecystectomy or those who are at high risk for surgery may be tried on ursodeoxycholic acid. Patients with evidence of choledocholithiasis (Figure 13-1) should undergo ERCP for removal of stones. In addition, any patient who has suffered complications from stone disease (pancreatitis, gallstone ileus, cholangitis) should undergo cholecystectomy when clinically stable.

## PEARLS/PITFALLS

- Patients being considered for elective cholecystectomy should have further evaluation for choledocholithiasis if liver enzyme abnormalities are noted and/or common bile duct dilation is noted on routine ultrasound.
- If the index of suspicion for choledocholithiasis is low-medium, an MRCP or EUS should be performed prior to ERCP.
- Do not rush to perform ERCP on a patient with active gallstone pancreatitis, unless cholangitis develops.

# Biliary Strictures

## PRESENTATION

Part of the workup of abnormal liver tests includes basic imaging to rule out anatomic abnormalities. Biliary strictures are often identified in this setting. Strictures can cause jaundice and occasional pain and can be the cause of cholangitis.

The etiology of biliary strictures can be infectious, malignant, autoimmune, inflammatory, or extrinsic causes. An adequate history will often help provide clues into the cause. For example, a patient with painless jaundice, weight loss, and imaging suggestive of ductal obstruction should immediately suggest a workup for pancreatic cancer. Primary sclerosis cholangitis should be suspected in a patient with ulcerative colitis who develops jaundice, elevated levels of alkaline phosphatase, and imaging suggestive of multifocal stricturing and dilations of intrahepatic and extrahepatic bile ducts.

## LAB STUDIES

Studies often reveal an elevation in alkaline phosphatase and total bilirubin. Additional laboratory studies may be obtained to help aid in the diagnosis of the underlying cause of the stricture/obstruction (ie, carbohydrate antigen 19-9, human immunodeficiency virus test, perinuclear anti-neutrophil cytoplasmic antibodies [P-ANCA], serum immunoglobulin G4 levels).

## IMAGING CHARACTERISTICS

Cholangiography is the test of choice to help delineate the cause of extent of biliary disease. MRCP is a useful test to help determine the cause and extent of biliary obstruction. In addition, it may help to determine if further invasive testing is needed like treatment of a dominant stricture or removal of an obstructive stone. ERCP should be performed when invasive diagnostic testing or therapeutic intervention is required. It will allow for brushing, biopsy, direct cholangioscopy, intraductal endoscopic ultrasound (IDUS), and stenting of obstructive strictures.

## MANAGEMENT

The treatment of obstructive jaundice from biliary strictures greatly depends on the etiology of the stricture and the symptoms. Benign strictures (ie, postsurgical) will often improve with dilation and stenting via ERCP. Presumed malignant strictures can be sampled via brushing,

**Figure 13-2.** ERCP showing
a hilar stricture with dilation
of intrahepatic ducts.

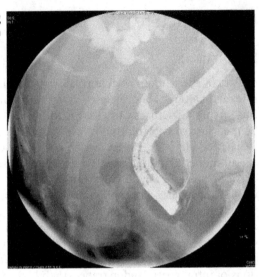

intraductal biopsy, and stented with ERCP. Figure 13-2 reveals a hilar
stricture. Some conditions, such as primary sclerosing cholangitis, are
more controversial and are usually not treated with ERCP unless there
is concern for underlying malignancy, cholangitis, or a dominant stricture. Cholangiocarcinoma can be difficult to diagnose, and ERCP with
cholangioscopy may aid in tissue acquisition. Concurrent biliary drainage can be performed, but care should be taken to drain all segments
of the liver into which contrast may have been injected to avoid severe
cholangitis.

## PEARLS/PITFALLS

- Brushings and biopsies alone have high specificity and low sensi-
  tivity, thus they should not be used alone to rule out malignancy.
  Direct cholangioscopy and IDUS are newer techniques that help
  improve yield.
- Jaundice (unless causing pruritus) alone is not a reason to perform
  ERCP.

# Choledochal Cysts

Choledochal cysts are cysts within the bile ducts.

## PRESENTATION

Most patients are asymptomatic. They may present with intermittent, vague abdominal pain, and routine imaging may subsequently

reveal the presence of a biliary cyst(s). Rarely, patients can present with jaundice or a palpable abdominal mass. These cysts are thought to be congenital, although there is some evidence that certain cysts may be acquired. Therefore, it is not uncommon for patients with biliary cysts to give a history of long-standing intermittent pain since childhood. In severe cases, children can develop severe obstructive jaundice and failure to thrive from biliary cysts. In addition, there is an association of biliary cysts with abnormal pancreatobiliary junction (ABPJ).

## CLASSIFICATION

- Type I: Cystic dilation of common bile duct (CBD); most common.
- Type II: Cystic outpouching or diverticulum of extrahepatic bile duct.
- Type III: Choledochocoele: cystic dilation of duodenal portion of distal common bile duct.
- Type IVA: Multiple cysts involving both intrahepatic and extrahepatic ducts.
- Type IVB: Multiple cysts involving only extrahepatic ducts.
- Type V: Multiple cysts within intrahepatic biliary ducts.

## LAB STUDIES

There are no specific laboratory abnormalities for biliary cysts. Patients may have laboratory results suggestive of biliary obstruction depending upon the severity of their cystic disease. It is not uncommon for patients to have elevated alkaline phosphatase and total bilirubin.

## IMAGING CHARACTERISTICS

The usual initial study, which might suggest the presence of a biliary cyst, is a transabdominal ultrasound or CT scan. The gold standard requires cholangiography. Noninvasive cholangiography can be obtained with MRCP, and this test is very useful for determining extent and location for biliary dilation. An EUS may be used to evaluate the area of dilation, focal bile duct wall thickening, and any intraductal abnormalities but is limited in its ability to evaluate the intrahepatic biliary system. Finally, ERCP is available for the diagnosis and classification of biliary cysts. The most useful benefit of ERCP is that it helps to definitively exclude biliary obstruction and can treat a particular type of biliary cyst (Type III).

**Figure 13-3.** Endoscopic view showing a Type III choledochal cyst (choledochocoele).

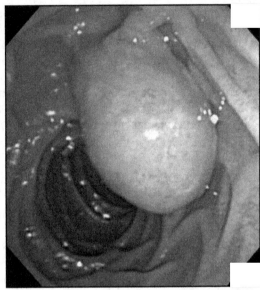

## MANAGEMENT

Aside from intermittent abdominal pain and jaundice, biliary cysts increase a patient's risk of developing cholangicarcinoma. Cystic lesions of the biliary system must be treated definitively, when possible, to reduce the risk of subsequent malignancy. The treatment is surgical, with the goal to remove all cysts if possible. Surgery may require extensive biliary reconstruction in some cases. The only form of biliary cyst that may be managed without surgery is the Type III choledochocoele, which can often be treated with ERCP and sphincteromy alone (Figure 13-3). The presence of anomalies of the pancreaticobiliary junction (APBJ) can make operative management more difficult, because the surgeon may be forced to remove part of the pancreas and/or require future endoscopic therapies.

## PEARLS/PITFALLS

- Not all dilations of the CBD are Type I cysts. Obstruction can lead to dilation of CBD and is not related to a true biliary cyst.
- If you are not sure if you are dealing with chronic dilation or a true cyst, look for APBJ to help make an accurate diagnosis.

- One is not done following patients after they have been referred for surgery. Patients can have repeat biliary obstruction from post-operative strictures and/or develop cancer. Follow these patients with routine labs and have a low threshold to image the abdomen if old or new symptoms occur.

- APBJ alone without biliary cyst increases risk of gallbladder cancer and is an indication for cholecystectomy.

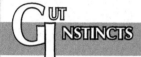

**GUT INSTINCTS** BILIARY DISEASES

1. Approximately 10% to 20% of severe acute cholecystitis cases are from acalculous cholecystitis, especially in the sick and elderly.
2. Patients being considered for elective cholecystectomy should have further evaluation for choledocholithiasis if liver enzyme abnormalities are noted and/or common bile duct dilation is noted on routine ultrasound.
3. If the index of suspicion for choledocholithiasis is low-medium, a MRCP or EUS should be performed prior to ERCP.
4. Brushings and biopsies alone have high specificity and low sensitivity for bile duct malignancy and should not be used alone to rule out malignancy.
5. Not all dilations of the CBD are Type I cysts. Obstruction can lead to dilation of CBD and is not related to a true biliary cyst.

## Key References

1. Huffman JL, Schenker S. Acute acalculous cholecystitis: a review. *Clin Gastroenterol Hepatol*. 2010;8(1):15-22.
2. O'Neill DE, Saunders MD. Endoscopic ultrasonography in diseases of the gallbladder. *Gastroenterol Clin North Am*. 2010;39(2):289-305, ix.

# CHAPTER 14

# CELIAC DISEASE

Wilfred M. Weinstein, MD

This chapter takes a "just the facts" approach to the most important aspects of the diagnosis and management of celiac disease. There are two diagnostic criteria: (1) a severe "flat" (Marsh 3) lesion exhibiting villous atrophy of the small intestinal mucosa; and (2) a clinical, biochemical (and histological) response to a gluten-free diet.

## Pathology and Pathogenesis

Gluten is the wheat protein of wheat, barley, and rye. Gliadin is an alcohol-soluble fraction of gluten that contains most of the toxic components. The "flat" histological lesion has absent villi and increased numbers of inflammatory cells. T-cells dominate the immune-mediated response. The small bowel mucosa is most severely affected proximally. The terminal ileum is usually normal. The disease may have been present since childhood, totally silent or clinically occult, and then become manifest later in life with presumed extension of the injury beyond the most proximal small intestine.

## The Presentations

This disease was considered a European disease, described in Dutch children after World War II, and then in adults in the early 1950s. Why the delayed realization of prevalence in the United States—the "Bruce Springsteen phenomenon"? Conditions described elsewhere, not "Born in the USA," often take years or decades to cross the oceans or

Esrailian E. *Gut Instincts: A Clinician's Handbook of Digestive and Liver Diseases* (pp 95-100).
© 2012 Taylor & Francis Group

| Table 14-1 | Celiac Disease: Nongastrointestinal Manifestations and Associated Disorders |
|---|---|

**The Nongastrointestinal Manifestations of Celiac Disease**

- Anemia
- Hyposplenism: Howell-Jolly bodies
- Short stature in children
- Osteopenia
- Hypertransaminasemia and fatty liver
- Infertility/miscarriages
- Aphthous stomatitis
- Epilepsy (occipital lobe)
- Polyneuropathy

| Associated Disorders | Prevalence |
|---|---|
| Immunoglobulin A deficiency | 2% to 3% |
| Dermatitis herpetiformis | 80+% |
| Primary biliary cirrhosis | 6% |
| Autoimmune hepatitis | 5% |
| Type 1 diabetes | 3% to 7% |
| Autoimmune thyroiditis | 3% to 5% |
| Down syndrome | 10% |
| Collagenous or lymphocytic colitis | Exact prevalence of symptomatic cases unknown |

hemispheres before they are seen as relevant in the United States. One in 100 to 200 individuals of White origin have the disease. This group has the highest prevalence. Many other races have celiac disease, but the exact prevalences are unknown. In some series, 25% of newly diagnosed celiacs are in their 70s.

Only 30% to 40% of patients present with overt symptoms: painless diarrhea, pale stools, weight loss, abdominal distension, and/or abdominal pain. The remainder present with the nongastrointestinal (GI) manifestations (Table 14-1). Not surprisingly, celiac disease may be buried in groups of patients with irritable bowel syndrome (IBS).

The mucosal injury is primarily in the proximal small intestine. The manifestations are malabsorption of iron, folic acid, calcium, and fat-soluble vitamins. Anemia and osteopenia are common isolated (monosymptomatic) deficiencies of specific nutrients, especially iron, and may be present.

The medical history and/or one or more non-GI manifestations (see Table 14-1) trigger suspicion. Celiac disease may occur in 10% of first-degree relatives and can be diagnosed in the course of screening first-degree relatives. Celiac disease may be found incidentally at endoscopy or in the course of an endoscopic evaluation for iron deficiency anemia. Small bowel biopsies are taken in this setting, and biopsies both from the duodenal bulb and from the proximal duodenum (at least 4 biopsies) should be taken.

Key clues from the medical history include the following:

• Unexplained anemia, most often iron deficiency.

• Shorter than same sex parent or sibling.

• Relative hyperphagia, eating more than one's weight would belie.

• Past unexplained weight loss and/or pale stools.

• Osteopenia is common in celiac disease. Diminished bone density is associated with an increased risk of fractures.

# Diagnosis

Serologic testing is the primary method for screening and diagnosis. Endomysial antibody (immunoglobin A [IgA]-EMA), tissue transglutaminase antibody (IgA-tTG), and a serum IgA are recommended because of the possibility of selective IgA deficiency. Human leukocyte antigen (HLA)-DQ2 and HLA-DQ8 are recommended for some complex cases. Antibodies against gliadin (IgA antiendomysial antibodies [IgA-AGA], immunoglobulin G-anti-gliadin antibodies [AGA]) have generally not been useful except for the newer deamidated forms.

Sensitivity for serologies is 90% to 95%. Serologic screening has revolutionized the approach to diagnosis and has uncovered those with "monosymptomatic" clinically occult features. As seen in Table 14-1, 2.5% of patients with celiac disease have selective IgA deficiency. This percentage is 10 to 15 times its prevalence in the general population. Immunoglobulin A levels should be obtained at the same time as the EMA and tTG. If IgA deficiency is present, an immunoglobin M (IgM)-based tTG is done. The patient with selective IgA deficiency should be alerted to tell physicians he or she has it in the event that other antibody tests are performed. HLA-DQ2 and/or HLA-DQ8 are present in all with celiac disease. By themselves, HLA do not point to the diagnosis. Instead, in less-straightforward cases, their absence rules out celiac disease.

The definitive first step in diagnosis is a "flat" avillous duodenal mucosa. The second step in diagnosis is a response to a gluten-free diet. Some seropositive patients have minimal lesions. Diarrhea attributed to minimal lesions is hard to accept except if it is associated with lactase deficiency. The implications of seropositive-associated minimal lesions or normal mucosa are unclear.

## Associated Disorders

Table 14-1 lists some of the disorders associated with celiac disease. The most important associations are Type 1 diabetes and autoimmune (Hashimoto's) thyroiditis. Routine screening for celiac disease in these disorders, especially in Type 1 diabetes and Hashimoto's thyroiditis, makes sense.

Dermatitis herpetiformis (DH) is an intensely pruritic vesiculobullous skin rash. At least 80% of individuals with DH have an intestinal biopsy indistinguishable from that of celiac disease. The skin disease improves completely with a gluten-free diet.

## Treatment and Prognosis

Therapy is gluten-free diet for life: no wheat, barley, or rye. There is now an ever-larger availability of gluten-free foods in stores. Few dieticians are familiar with the practical aspects and nuances of the gluten-free diet. Celiac support groups are the best source of information. Gluten or wheat flour is often used as filler in processed foods and in cooking foods, such as scrambled eggs and hamburgers. The best rule of thumb in eating out is, "if anything could come between the plants or the fish/meat and you, don't eat it, keep it simple."

In patients with diarrhea, a lactose-free diet may help in its own right because there is commonly secondary lactase deficiency. Mucosal lactase returns within 1 or 2 months on the gluten-free diet, and lactose can be reintroduced after some time to see if lactose is tolerated.

Patients should not empirically start a gluten-free diet because they may fail to respond in bona fide celiac disease for various reasons and some real responders do not have celiac disease as it is known. Response without biopsy means gluten-free diet for life and screening relatives. If such patients agree to a biopsy diagnosis, they need a gluten challenge for several months or until symptoms appear.

The vast majority of patients have a good response to a gluten-free diet. Those who do not may have inadvertent gluten ingestion or other conditions as the basis of the abnormal mucosa, such as common variable immunodeficiency and small intestinal bacterial overgrowth. A small percentage has refractory or unclassified sprue.

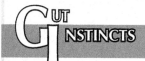

GUT GI INSTINCTS                                         CELIAC DISEASE

1. Celiac disease is common. Keep a list nearby of GI, non-GI manifestations, and associated disorders.

2. Only 30% to 40% of patients have diarrhea/steatorrhea.

3. Serology is important when celiac disease is suspected on the basis of GI or non-GI manifestations.

4. Check for serum IgA deficiency to help with interpretation of serologies and to avoid false negatives.

5. Biopsy, and not an empiric trial of a gluten-free diet, is the definitive first step.

# Key References

1. Green PH, Cellier C. Celiac disease. *N Engl J Med*. 2007;25;357(17):1731-1743.
2. Rubio-Tapia A, Murray JA. Celiac disease. *Curr Opin Gastroenterol*. 2010;26(2):116-122.
3. Tack GJ, Verbeek WH, Schreurs MW, Mulder CJ. The spectrum of celiac disease: epidemiology, clinical aspects and treatment. *Nat Rev Gastroenterol Hepatol*. 2010;7(4):204-213.

# CHAPTER 15

# BARIATRIC SURGERY PATIENTS

Erik P. Dutson, MD, FACS and
David Da Zheng, BS

Postoperative bariatric patients represent a unique challenge for evaluation and care, due to their anatomic alterations, physiological state, and tendency to decompensate rapidly in the early postoperative period. With morbid obesity affecting a startling and growing percent of the US population and bariatric surgeries numbering more than 200,000/year, familiarity with this patient population is essential for the safe practice of gastroenterology. The 2 most common procedures performed in the United States are laparoscopic adjustable gastric band (LAGB) and Roux-en-Y gastric bypass (RYGB). This chapter uses an outline form to highlight important complications and management options for the practicing clinician.

## Laparoscopic Adjustable Gastric Band

LAGB is an inflatable, synthetic band placed around the stomach just below the gastroesophageal junction. It can be deflated or inflated through a subcutaneous port to regulate the passage of food.

### Surgical Complications

#### Band Slippage (Incidence: ~5%)

Slippage of gastric tissue through the band may be irregular and slight, or it may be severe and may not resolve. Gastric necrosis may result.

Esrailian E. *Gut Instincts: A Clinician's Handbook of Digestive and Liver Diseases* (pp 101-108).

- Symptoms include acute nausea, intolerance of liquids or foods, and vomiting.
- Diagnosis: Upper gastrointestinal (UGI) series or computed tomography (CT) with oral contrast can confirm band slippage.
- Treatment: For a mild slip, deflate band, and reassess in 1 to 2 weeks. For a moderate slip, deflate and surgically reposition versus revision. For a severe slip, deflate, and surgically remove.

### Gastric Erosion (Incidence: <2% of cases)

Erosion is migration of the band through the gastric wall. Erosion can manifest as erythema or cellulitis at the skin over port site and mandates investigation for erosion. It can also manifest as port leak if the balloon ruptures.

- Symptoms include pain, erythema, and swelling at the port site. With a full-thickness erosion, restriction is lost. The patient will notice an ability to eat more.
- Diagnostic studies: UGI can show evidence of intraluminal band position, and an upper endoscopy is definitive.
- Treatment: An erosion is rarely an emergency. If the access port site is infected, surgical removal is indicated to treat infection. Alternatively, if a portion of the band is visible by endoscopy, it can be divided and endoscopically removed in piecemeal fashion with snare/cautery.

### Esophageal Dysmotility

LAGB has been associated with esophageal dysfunction. Gastroesophageal reflux disease (GERD) and esophagitis may result in permanent stricture or dilation of the esophagus.

- Symptoms include chronic heartburn, dysphagia, and regurgitation.
- Diagnostic studies: UGI can be used for the evaluation of stricture/gastric outlet obstruction and esophageal diameter. Ambulatory pH monitoring can evaluate for GERD. Esophageal manometry is used to assess for dysmotility/megaesophagus. Upper endoscopy can diagnose Barrett's esophagus and esophageal strictures, which can be dilated during the procedure.
- Treatment: Over-the-counter antacids can be used for temporary relief in addition to histamine-2-receptor antagonists (H2RA) and proton pump inhibitors (PPIs) for maintenance therapy. If there is evidence of esophageal dysmotility, Barrett's esophagus, or gastric outlet obstruction, surgical referral is indicated.

# Roux-en-Y Gastric Bypass

In the RYGB, a 15- to 30-mL gastric pouch is created, which is anastomosed to the jejunum. The jejunojejunostomy is created between 75 and 100 cm distal, which defines the actual bypassed segment of the stomach and the proximal small bowel. Upper gastrointestinal bleeding and marginal ulcers are the most common complications, with an incidence approximating 5%.

## SURGICAL COMPLICATIONS

### Anastomotic Leak, Potentially Lethal (Incidence: 1%)

Risk factors include older patients, males with multiple comorbidities, and a body mass index (BMI) >50.

- Symptoms include sustained tachycardia >120 bpm, tachypnea, and fever. In addition, patient may have chest pain, dyspnea, anxiety, arrhythmias, and abdominal pain.
- Diagnostic studies: UGI with gastrografin, not barium, should be used. A CT scan with both intravenous (IV) and oral contrast has the highest yield.
- Treatment: A suspected leak should lead to immediate surgical referral. Surgery involves washout, repair, and drain placement.

### Obstruction/Internal Hernia (Possibly Lethal)

- Symptoms include intermittent, postprandial abdominal pain. There may also be bloating, persistent hiccups, nausea, vomiting, and acute pain.
- Diagnostic studies: CT findings suggestive of internal hernia include small bowel loops in the left upper quadrant and a "swirl sign," indicative of volvulized mesentery; UGI reveals a closed loop obstruction and no passage of contrast beyond a certain point.
- Treatment: Partial obstruction may resolve without surgical intervention, but eventual exploration is still indicated. A nasogastric tube (NGT) must only be placed under fluoroscopy. Complete obstruction will require surgical intervention. The index of suspicion must be high for early detection to reduce morbidity and mortality.

### Stomal Stenosis (Incidence: Up to 15%)

- Symptoms include postprandial regurgitation, vomiting, and epigastric pain. Patients may be intolerant to liquids, and even saliva, in severe cases.
- Diagnostic studies: UGI can identify gastrojejunal stenosis or stricture.
- Treatment: Endoscopic stomal dilatation can be performed, but should not exceed 15-mm diameter due to risk of disrupting the anastomosis or causing loss of its restrictive function.

### Acute Gastric Remnant Dilatation

- Symptoms include left upper quadrant pain, persistent tachycardia, and hiccups.
- Diagnostic studies: CT is used to identify a cause, such as distal obstruction.
- Treatment: Gastrostomy tube decompression is used for chronic dilatation. Surgical revision of the jejunojejunostomy is indicated for acute dilatation.

### Stomal Ulcer (Incidence: 3% to 8%)

- Symptoms include retrosternal or epigastric pain, dyspepsia, and vomiting.
- Diagnostic studies: Endoscopy is the gold standard, and biopsies can be taken for *Helicobacter pylori*.
- Treatment: *H. pylori* can be treated through standard triple antibiotic therapy. PPIs daily or twice daily and sucralfate slurry can be used in combination. Patients should eliminate smoking, alcohol, and nonsteroidal anti-inflammatory drugs.

## NUTRITIONAL COMPLICATIONS

### General Malnutrition

- Symptoms include malabsorption and severe weight loss beyond what would be expected after surgery. Patients may have an emaciated appearance and temporal wasting.
- Diagnostic laboratory tests: Low protein, fat, and vitamin levels (see p. 106).
- Treatment: 1500 Kcal/day diet, 80 to 100 g protein/day, multivitamin (MVI), calcium, sublingual vitamin $B_{12}$, and possibly iron.

### Dumping Syndrome

Dumping is usually caused by dietary noncompliance.

- Symptoms include diarrhea, abdominal cramps, nausea, and vomiting. Systemic manifestations include hypotension, tachycardia, flushing, lightheadedness, and syncope.
- Prevention: Dumping can be minimized by avoiding refined carbohydrates and eating more slowly.

### Iron Deficiency

The primary sites of absorption are bypassed with RYGB. In addition, many patients often have a poor tolerance of red meat. Premenopausal women are more vulnerable.

- Presentation: Many patients present only with microcytic anemia.
- Diagnostic laboratory tests: Complete blood count (CBC) and iron panels are often diagnostic. A serum iron, transferrin, and ferritin should be checked semiannually.
- Treatment: Oral ferrous sulfate, 325 mg/day, may be effective if taken between meals with vitamin C. Iron-rich foods are encouraged. However, because of malabsorption, many patients require intramuscular (IM) iron injections or parenteral IV iron.

### Folic Acid Deficiency

- Symptoms: Folate deficiency can present with megaloblastic anemia, glossitis, and leukopenia. In pregnancy, it may result in neural tube defects.
- Diagnostic laboratory tests: Routine serum folate levels and CBC are used to determine if supplementation is needed.
- Treatment: Supplementation with folate 1 mg/day is usually adequate.

### Vitamin $B_{12}$ Deficiency

- Symptoms: Megaloblastic anemia, leukopenia, glossitis, thrombocytopenia, and irreversible neural demyelination can develop.
- Diagnostic laboratory test: A vitamin $B_{12}$ level should be checked.
- Treatment: Daily sublingual $B_{12}$ versus weekly IM injections are used.

### Vitamin D Deficiency

- Symptoms: Osteomalacia, recurrent metabolic syndrome, and muscle cramps/aches can develop.
- Prevention: Daily vitamin D supplements of 400 to 2000 IU/d are used.

*Thiamine Deficiency*

- Symptoms: Wernicke-Korsakoff syndrome can develop with confusion and psychosis, and it can be preceded by vomiting and rapid weight loss. Dry beriberi presents with symmetric impairment of sensory, motor, and reflex functions. Wet beriberi presents with mental confusion, muscular wasting, edema, and tachycardia.
- Diagnostic laboratory test: Thiamine level should be checked in every postbariatric patient because deficiency is common from noncompliance and commonly presents with an odd constellation of symptoms.
- Treatment: Daily MVI is usually sufficient for prevention, and 50 mg IV/IM should correct the deficiency if needed.

*Calcium Deficiency*

- Symptoms: The presentations can vary but include osteoporosis, perioral tingling and parasthesia, laryngospasm, and cardiac arrhythmias.
- Diagnostic laboratory test: Serum calcium levels should be followed.
- Prevention: Routine oral supplementation (1500 to 2000 mg/d) is recommended. All postbariatric patients should take calcium supplements daily.

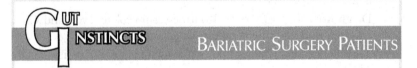

GUT INSTINCTS                          BARIATRIC SURGERY PATIENTS

1. Always check/give thiamine in RYGB patients.
2. No nasogastric tubes should be placed without fluoroscopy.
3. Use extreme caution during endoscopy immediately distal to the gastroesophageal junction.
4. CT scan of the abdomen is generally the best diagnostic test.
5. Clinicians should have a high index of suspicion for internal hernia in patients with postprandial pain after RYGB.

# Key References

1. Belle SH, Berk PD, Courcoulas AP, et al; Longitudinal Assessment of Bariatric Surgery Consortium Writing Group. Safety and efficacy of bariatric surgery: longitudinal assessment of bariatric surgery. *Surg Obes Relat Dis.* 2007;3(2):116-126.

2. Gamagaris Z, Patterson C, Schaye V, et al. Lap-band impact on the function of the esophagus. *Obes Surg.* 2008;18(10):1268-1272.

# LOWER GASTROINTESTINAL TRACT

# CHAPTER 16

# ULCERATIVE COLITIS

Gil Y. Melmed, MD, MS

Ulcerative colitis (UC) represents chronic inflammation involving the colon. Symptoms usually correspond to the disease severity. Milder symptoms may be limited to sporadic blood seen in the stool, while more severe symptoms can include frank hematochezia with diarrhea, often accompanied by tenesmus and lower abdominal pain on the left side. In fulminant UC, patients may have more than 10 bowel movements daily accompanied by systemic signs or symptoms of toxicity including fever, severe abdominal pain, and even hemodynamic instability. Historically, fulminant UC carried significant mortality due to the high risk of spontaneous perforation and sepsis. Nowadays, UC is not a fatal condition due to the use of immunosuppressive therapies and timely surgical intervention.

## Diagnosis

UC is characterized by mucosal inflammation that begins distally, in the rectum, and involves some or all of the more proximal colonic mucosa in a continuous, diffuse pattern. It can be difficult to distinguish between UC and Crohn's disease limited to the colon. Endoscopically, the inflammation of UC typically appears shallow, without deeper serpiginous or linear ulcers characteristic of Crohn's disease. Backwash ileitis refers to mild ileal inflammation involving only a few centimeters of terminal ileum, thought to result from reflux of the inflammatory effluent into the ileum from the proximal colon. However, ileal

Esrailian E. *Gut Instincts: A Clinician's Handbook of Digestive and Liver Diseases* (pp 111-116).

inflammation of greater extent or with discrete ulceration(s) likely represents Crohn's disease. Therefore, colonoscopy with ileal evaluation is critical for the diagnosis and classification of colonic inflammation as either UC or Crohn's disease. Other useful tests to clarify the diagnosis of UC may include serologies (p-ANCA) and stool markers of inflammation (calprotectin or lactoferrin) which may help distinguish inflammatory from functional diarrhea.

## Treatment

It is important to characterize the extent and severity of UC to optimally target both the type of therapy and its mode of delivery. The treatment pyramid refers to the sequential use of potentially more toxic therapies for those with more severe or refractory symptoms (Figure 16-1). The 5-aminosalicylate (5-ASA) products (ie, mesalamine, balsalazide, sulfasalazine) are generally very safe and effective therapy for patients with mild to moderate UC. The effectiveness of 5-ASA products in UC is in apparent contradistinction from small bowel Crohn's disease, where 5-ASA products are generally not effective. 5-ASA can be delivered orally or topically to the site of distal colonic inflammation in the form of a suppository or enema. Therefore, it is critical to establish the extent of inflammation to target therapy.

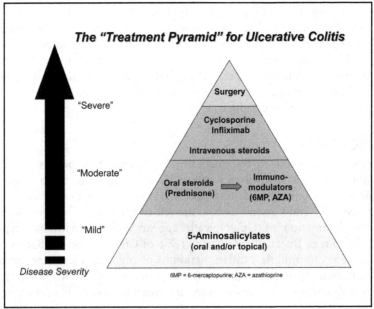

**Figure 16-1.** The "treatment pyramid" for UC.

Mesalamine suppositories can treat inflammation limited to the distal 10 cm of the colon, while enemas can deliver medication to inflammation extending up to the splenic flexure. A combination of oral and topical therapy is more effective than either modality alone for patients with left-sided colonic inflammation. However, symptoms of rectal inflammation (tenesmus and bowel frequency due to poor rectal distensibility) can be treated with topical therapy even for those with more extensive pancolitis (involving most or all of the colon). Reduction in inflammation in the very distal colon can significantly improve symptoms even in the setting of more proximal inflammation. Patients with mild to moderate UC will usually experience symptom improvement within 2 weeks after initiating mesalamine therapy at an appropriate dose. Once complete symptom improvement (remission) has been achieved, patients should maintain therapy on a regular dose of 5-ASA (oral and/or topical) to reduce the risk of recurrence.

## Moderate to Severe Colitis

Moderate to severe UC may not respond to 5-ASA alone and may require immunosuppressive treatment to induce and/or maintain remission. Traditionally, steroids have been prescribed in this setting, usually at 40 mg of prednisone daily, followed by a taper once symptoms are improved. Patients can be induced with steroids and maintained on 5-ASA products, although some patients may require retreatment with steroids for disease recurrence despite 5-ASA treatment. Those requiring 2 or more courses of prednisone may benefit from long-term immunosuppressive therapy with immunomodulators (6-mercaptopurine, azathioprine) or infliximab. Some patients may become steroid dependent, and others may become steroid refractory, where steroids are not effective at controlling symptoms. Either way, escalation of therapy (assuming the symptoms are due to UC and not an enteric infection such as *Clostridium difficile*) is appropriate. Steroid-dependent patients can be transitioned onto immunomodulators and/or infliximab. Steroid-refractory disease in the stable outpatient can be treated with infliximab or may warrant admission to the hospital for intravenous steroids and further evaluation.

Patients needing hospitalization should undergo stool testing for *C. difficile* and should be considered for a sigmoidoscopy with biopsies to assess for cytomegalovirus. Those refractory to outpatient oral steroids should be treated with intravenous corticosteroids; doses higher than the equivalent of 60 mg methylprednisolone (divided 3 times daily) are not associated with better outcomes, but increase the risk of adverse effects. Hospitalized patients with UC should undergo careful daily abdominal examination to assess for megacolon and signs of peritonitis, which can be masked by steroids and narcotics. They should receive prophylaxis against thromboembolism with subcutaneous heparin, even if ambulatory, given increased risks of venous thromboembolic events in this population.

Surgical consultation should be obtained early because patients who are not clinically improved by days 3 to 5 of intravenous steroids should be considered for cyclosporine, infliximab, or colectomy. Those with signs of systemic toxicity should go straight to surgery to reduce the risk of morbidity and mortality. Intravenous cyclosporine can reduce the short-term risk of colectomy by 70%, but at 1 year, the colectomy-free rate is about 50% and continues to decrease over time. Infliximab may also reduce the rate of colectomy in the short term and can be used for maintenance after hospitalization. However, cyclosporine should not be administered shortly after infliximab administration due to significant infectious risks. If surgery is being considered, patients will generally be presented with the option of a total proctocolectomy with an end ileostomy (Brooke ileostomy), or an ileal pouch-anal anastomosis (IPAA), which allows for preservation of sphincter continence. If an adequate small bowel evaluation has previously not been performed, a small bowel imaging test (computed tomography/magnetic resonance enterography or barium small-bowel series) should be performed to clarify whether there is evidence of small bowel disease that would preclude creation of an ileal pouch. Inflammatory bowel disease (IBD)-specific serologies can also help to prognosticate outcomes after surgery because patients with elevated anti-*Saccharomyces cerevisiae* antibodies immunoglobulin A may have a higher risk of pouch complications including the *de novo* development of Crohn's disease in the ileal pouch.

# Health Care Maintenance of the Patient With Ulcerative Colitis

Patients with UC should be seen regularly by their gastroenterologists, even when in remission due to the need for ongoing health care maintenance. The risk of colon cancer significantly increases with the duration of UC. After 8 years of disease, patients should undergo surveillance colonoscopies for dysplasia with random biopsies every 1 to 3 years, with the interval determined by overall cancer risk, which increases with greater extent and duration of disease, family history of colon cancer, and having primary sclerosing cholangitis. Patients with inflammatory bowel disease may be at risk for bone demineralization, either from the disease itself or from steroid exposure. Therefore, patients should be referred for bone densitometry, especially if exposed to steroids, and may require supplementation with calcium and vitamin D. Finally, patients should be educated regarding the risks of vaccine-preventable infections because immunosuppressive medications may increase the risk of these infections and render immunizations less effective. In particular, consideration for influenza and pneumococcal vaccinations are appropriate for all patients with IBD regardless of their immunosuppressed status.

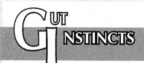

## ULCERATIVE COLITIS

1. Patients with a new diagnosis of UC should have a full colonoscopy to determine the extent and severity of disease to target treatment.

2. UC requires ongoing maintenance therapy even in the absence of symptoms once remission has been achieved.

3. Patients with a severe flare of UC should be assessed for *Clostridium difficile* infection.

4. Those with UC not responding to an adequate course of steroid therapy (eg, steroid equivalent of prednisone 40 mg daily for 10 days) should be hospitalized for further evaluation and treatment.

5. Those with UC should be educated about the risks of colon cancer and begin a dysplasia surveillance program after having the disease for 8 to 10 years.

## Key References

1. Long MD, Plevy SE. Poorly responsive ulcerative colitis in the hospital. *Clin Gastroenterol Hepatol.* 2009;7(6):635-640.

2. Baumgart DC, Sandborn WJ. Inflammatory bowel disease: clinical aspects and established and evolving therapies. *Lancet.* 2007;369(9573):1641-1657.

3. Kornbluth A, Sachar DB, Practice Parameters Committee of the American College of Gastroenterology. Ulcerative colitis practice guidelines in adults: American College of Gastroenterology, Practice Parameters Committee. *Am J Gastroenterol.* 2010;105(3):501-523.

# CHAPTER 17

# CROHN'S DISEASE

Marla Dubinsky, MD

Crohn's disease (CD) is characterized by chronic intestinal inflammation. The exact etiology remains unclear; however, research continues to advance at a rapid pace to try and uncover the mysteries of this heterogeneous inflammatory process. Two important discoveries have been made in the past decade: the role of genetic susceptibility in CD and the introduction of monoclonal antibodies targeted to tumor-necrosis factor alpha (TNFα). This chapter will highlight advances in the diagnosis and management of CD and how genetics is shaping the individualization of treatment approaches.

## Epidemiology and Etiology

CD, especially in the pediatric age group, has increased in prevalence in the past decade. There does not appear to be gender predominance, and the emerging pattern suggests similar patterns of disease incidence in Whites and non-Whites, those who live in urban and those who live in rural areas, and those in more northern and southern latitudes. Ashkenazi Jewish background appears to be a risk factor, as does a family history. Environmental factors such as improved living conditions early in life increase the likelihood of developing CD.

Although the etiology is unclear, CD is thought to result from a complex interaction of genetic, host immune, and environmental factors. The single greatest risk factor for the development of inflammatory bowel disease (IBD) is having a first-degree relative with the condition,

Esrailian E. *Gut Instincts: A Clinician's Handbook of Digestive and Liver Diseases* (pp 117-122).

with the estimated risk 30 to 100 times greater than in the general population. At the time of diagnosis of CD, the likelihood of finding IBD in a first-degree relative of the proband is 10% to 25%. Through the use of genome-wide association study analyses, the number of susceptibility loci associated with CD has grown exponentially. Nucleotide-binding oligomerization domain containing 2 (NOD2) was the first CD susceptibility gene identified in 2001. Since then, there have been approximately 70 CD susceptibility genes identified, and a recent meta-analysis uncovered a number of ulcerative colitis (UC) genes. The idea that IBD is a spectrum of diseases rather than simply classified as either CD or UC was brought to the forefront when many gene loci were found in both CD and UC patients. To date, no pathogen has reproducibly been identified as a potential cause of CD. A complex interaction of gut mucosal immune mechanisms with intestinal flora, however, is thought to be critical in the development of CD. This interaction may allow increased permeability to bacterial or other antigens, leading to unchecked stimulation of local immune cells. The abnormal immune response may be a result of defective barrier function or, alternatively, defective downregulation of an appropriate response to luminal stimulation.

## Clinical Features and Diagnosis

Patients with CD classically present with abdominal pain, change in consistency and frequency of bowel movements, weight loss, and fatigue. Despite the classic symptoms, clinical presentations may also vary among individuals commonly driven by location of disease. For those 20% to 30% of patients with colon-predominate disease, their presentation overlaps more with those symptoms seen in patients with UC (rectal bleeding, urgency, frequency). A subgroup of patients with perianal disease will complain of anal pain and drainage in the face of fistulas and/or fissures. Patients with stricturing disease may complain of bloating, early satiety, and pain with eating, which are symptoms that merit an evaluation for possible small bowel obstruction.

The gold standard diagnostic workup includes colonoscopy and radiological evaluation with histologic confirmation of macroscopic findings. Small bowel involvement usually differentiates CD and UC, although patchy colonic disease may be the only presentation for Crohn's colitis. UC usually has a more contiguous disease, which also usually involves the rectum. Advances in small bowel imaging have improved the ability to detect active mucosal disease. Wireless capsule endoscopy and magnetic resonance enterography provide small bowel visualization without the risks of radiation that accompany computed tomography enterography and fluoroscopic-based tests.

| TABLE 17-1 | CONVENTIONAL CROHN'S DISEASE THERAPIES | |
|---|---|---|
| Treatment | Examples | Common Uses in CD* |
| Aminosalicylates (5-ASAs) | Mesalamine, Sulfasalazine | For first-line therapy for mild CD |
| Corticosteroids | Budesonide | For mild to moderate ileocecal CD |
| | Prednisone, Methylprednisolone | For moderate to severe CD |
| Antibiotics | Metronidazole, Ciprofloxacin | For perianal CD |
| | | For mild to moderate colonic CD |
| Immunosuppressants | Azathioprine, 6-Mercaptopurine, Methotrexate | For maintenance of a steroid-free remission |
| | | For perianal CD |
| CD indicates Crohn's disease | | |

## Treatment

Treatment of CD depends on disease location and the severity of disease (Table 17-1). The goals of therapy are to induce and maintain a steroid-free remission. Aminosalicylate preparations (5-ASA) are often prescribed for the induction and maintenance of remission but are the least effective CD anti-inflammatory therapies. There may be a role for 5-ASA drugs in colonic-predominant CD, but they are unlikely to have any role for small bowel CD. Antibiotics are also used to treat active disease, particularly colonic CD. Corticosteroids are sometimes needed on a short-term basis to induce remission. A newer corticosteroid, enteric-coated budesonide, has fewer systemic side effects and can be used to treat mild to moderate ileocolonic CD. Many CD patients require treatment with immunomodulators, such as azathioprine/6-mercaptopurine (6-MP) or methotrexate. Due to delayed onset of action, drugs in this class of medications are used as maintenance drugs and are useful in patients who have moderately active disease or steroid-dependent disease.

As noted above, the most significant advance in therapies for CD has been the introduction of biological therapies targeted to TNFα. Currently, 3 anti-TNFs are approved for induction and maintenance

| TABLE 17-2 | DOSING OF ANTI-TNFα THERAPIES | | | |
|---|---|---|---|---|
| Agent | Induction Dosing | Adult Maintenance Dose | Interval Between Maintenance Injections (Weeks) | Route |
| Infliximab | 5 mg/kg at 0, 2, and 6 weeks | 5 mg/kg (10 mg/kg in responders who lose response) | 8 | IV (over no less than 2 hours) |
| Adalimumab | 160 mg at week 0 followed by 80 mg at week 2 | 40 mg | 2 | SC |
| Certolizumab | 400 mg at 0, 2, and 4 weeks | 400 mg | 4 | SC |

of remission in CD: infliximab, adalimumab, and certolizumab pegol (Table 17-2). Although head-to-head studies have not been performed, all 3 appear to be similarly effective and have similar safety profiles. Combination immunomodulator and anti-TNFα has been shown to be superior to both azathioprine and infliximab monotherapy. However, the concern of lymphoma, more specifically hepatosplenic lymphoma, has not led to universal adoption of combination therapy in moderate to severe CD. Natalizumab, which targets adhesion molecules, represents an alternative class of therapies for CD. The risk of progressive multifocal leukoencephalopathy, however, precludes its widespread use and is limited to primary and secondary nonresponders to anti-TNFα. The risks and benefits of all therapies have become an important part of clinical decision making and must be weighed against the risk of undertreated or untreated disease. Surgery remains an important therapeutic option and can be considered in lieu of medical therapy or more commonly when medications have failed and a patient has experienced a complication such as stricturing or penetrating disease.

# Prognosis

Natural history studies suggest that close to 80% of patients will develop a complication, often necessitating surgery despite medical therapy. These data predate the regular and appropriate use of immunomodulators and the introduction of biologics. Follow-up studies do suggest that biologics reduce hospitalizations and surgeries in CD patients in the short term. Long-term studies are needed to determine if biologic therapies do, indeed, alter the natural history of CD. Biomarkers, as predictors of risk as well as in guiding therapy, are emerging as an important research area in CD and will help clinicians individualize therapies so the right therapy is being used for the right patient. Both genetics and serologic immune markers have been shown to stratify patients into those at risk for more rapid disease progression, helping identify the patients who will benefit from early effective intervention.

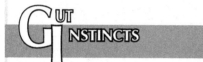

GUT INSTINCTS                                    CROHN'S DISEASE

1. Close to 70 genes have been identified for CD susceptibility, but these only account for 25% of the hereditability of CD.
2. Wireless capsule endoscopy and magnetic resonance enterography are useful tools to assess small bowel disease and to reduce the risk of radiation associated with computed tomography scans and traditional fluoroscopic examinations of the small bowel.
3. The 5-aminosalicylate drugs have a limited role in small bowel CD for induction or maintenance of disease remission.
4. Immunomodulators are effective for maintaining a steroid-free remission in patients with moderate disease.
5. Anti-TNF$\alpha$ therapies alone, and in combination with azathioprine, are effective for the induction and maintenance of remission in CD.

# Key References

1. Hanauer SB, Feagan BG, Lichtenstein GR, et al. Maintenance infliximab for Crohn's disease: the ACCENT I randomized trial. *Lancet.*
   2002;359(9317):1541-1549.
2. Colombel JF, Sandborn WJ, Reinisch W, et al. Infliximab, azathioprine,
   or combination therapy for Crohn's disease. *N Engl J Med.* 2010;362(15):
   1383-1395.
3. Dubinsky MC, Kugathasan S, Mei L, et al. Increased immune reactivity pre-
   dicts aggressive complicating Crohn's disease in children. *Clin Gastoenterol
   Hepatol.* 2008;6(10):1105-1111.

# CHAPTER 18

# POUCHITIS

Udayakumar Navaneethan, MD and
Bo Shen, MD, FACG

Approximately 30% of patients with ulcerative colitis (UC) eventually require colectomy at some point, despite advances in medical therapy. Restorative proctocolectomy with ileal pouch-anal anastomosis (IPAA) has become the surgical treatment of choice for the majority of patients with medically refractory UC, UC with dysplasia, or familial adenomatous polyposis. Pouchitis is a nonspecific inflammation of the ileal pouch reservoir and is the most frequent long-term complication of IPAA in patients with UC, with a cumulative prevalence of up to 50%.

## Classification of Pouchitis

There is not a uniform system for the classification of pouchitis. Pouchitis may be classified based on the etiology, disease duration and activity, and response to medical therapy into: (1) idiopathic versus secondary; (2) acute (<4 weeks) versus chronic (≥4 weeks); (3) infrequent episodes (<2 acute episodes) versus relapsing (≥3 acute episodes) versus continuous; and (4) antibiotic responsive versus refractory. Pouchitis can be classified based on the etiology into idiopathic and secondary pouchitis. Idiopathic pouchitis is believed to be triggered by dysbiosis leading to altered mucosal immune response in the majority of patients. Secondary pouchitis is defined as pouchitis with identifiable etiopathogenetic or triggering factors, and approximately 20% to 30% of patients with chronic antibiotic refractory pouchitis are estimated to have secondary causes.

Esrailian E. *Gut Instincts: A Clinician's Handbook of Digestive and Liver Diseases* (pp 123-128).
© 2012 Taylor & Francis Group

The various etiologies identified thus far include *Clostridium difficile* and other infections (infectious pouchitis), candida, cytomegalovirus, nonsteroidal anti-inflammatory drugs (NSAID)-induced pouchitis), collagen deposition of the pouch mucosa (collagenous pouchitis), ischemia (ischemic pouchitis), radiation injury (radiation pouchitis), chemotherapy (chemotherapy-associated pouchitis), concurrent autoimmune disorders (pouchitis associated with other autoimmune disorders), immunoglobulin G4-associated pouchopathy, and fecal diversion (diversion pouchitis).

Pouchitis can also be classified based on its response to antibiotics as antibiotic-responsive, antibiotic-dependent, and antibiotic-refractory pouchitis. Classification based on the response to antibiotic therapy is useful in clinical practice. Antibiotic-responsive pouchitis is characterized by infrequent episodes (fewer than 4 episodes per year) responding to a 2-week course of a single antibiotic. Antibiotic-dependent pouchitis is more challenging, and the patients often require long-term maintenance therapy to keep disease in remission. Patients have frequent episodes (4 or more episodes per year) of pouchitis or have persistent symptoms, which necessitate long term, continuous antibiotic or probiotic therapy. Chronic antibiotic-refractory pouchitis is defined as a condition in which a patient fails to respond to a 4-week course of a single antibiotic (metronidazole or ciprofloxacin) or requires prolonged therapy of 4 or more weeks consisting of 2 or more antibiotics, oral or topical 5-aminosalicylate, corticosteroid therapy, or an oral immunomodulator therapy.

## Diagnosis

Diagnosis of pouchitis is not always straightforward because there are no specific symptoms and signs. The usual presenting symptoms include increased stool frequency, urgency, incontinence, nocturnal seepage, abdominal cramps, and pelvic discomfort. Patients may occasionally present with extraintestinal manifestations such as arthralgias, jaundice, and pruritus from concomitant primary sclerosing cholangitis. However, these symptoms are not specific for pouchitis, and they can be present in other inflammatory and noninflammatory disorders of the pouch. In addition, severity of symptoms does not necessarily correlate with the degree of endoscopic or histologic inflammation of the pouch. Therefore, a combined assessment of symptoms and endoscopic and histologic features is advocated for the diagnosis and differential diagnosis of pouchitis. Various diagnostic criteria have been used, such as symptom assessment alone, symptom and endoscopy assessment (modified pouchitis disease activity index [mPDAI]), or symptom and endoscopy assessment with histology evaluation (PDAI), Heidelberg's criteria, and St. Marks' criteria. The PDAI score is the most common criteria used in research studies. A PDAI score greater than 7 suggests a diagnosis of pouchitis. In clinical practice, the diagnosis of pouchitis is ideally made based on the triad of compatible symptoms and endoscopic and histologic findings.

## Differential Diagnosis

A variety of inflammatory and noninflammatory disorders of the ileal pouch present with symptoms similar to pouchitis. Cuffitis is considered a variant form of UC in the rectal cuff, particularly in patients with IPAA without mucosectomy. Patients with cuffitis often present with bloody bowel movements, which rarely occur in pouchitis. The other common inflammatory disorder that mimics pouchitis is Crohn's disease (CD) of the pouch. IPAA surgery is speculated to create a "CD-friendly" environment with change of bowel anatomy, anastomoses, and fecal stasis. Although CD of the pouch can occur after IPAA in a selected group of patients with Crohn's colitis, *de novo* CD of the pouch is the most common form of CD and may develop weeks to years after IPAA for UC or indeterminate colitis. Clinical phenotypes of CD of the pouch can be inflammatory, fibrostenotic, or fistulizing. There are symptoms and signs suggesting a diagnosis of CD, particularly fibrostenotic and fistulizing CD. It is critical to differentiate NSAID-induced ileitis/pouchitis from CD ileitis. A diagnosis of CD of the pouch often needs a combined assessment of symptom, endoscopy, histology, radiography, and sometimes examination under anesthesia. Irritable pouch syndrome is a functional disorder in patients with IPAA. There is a great overlap in the clinical presentation between irritable pouch syndrome and pouchitis. Pouch endoscopy is the diagnostic modality of choice for the distinction between pouchitis and irritable pouch syndrome.

## Management

The management strategies vary based on different types of pouchitis. Because the majority of pouchitis is of bacterial etiology, antibiotic therapy is the primary therapy. Patients with a suspected diagnosis of acute pouchitis are usually started on metronidazole (15 to 20 mg/kg/day) or ciprofloxacin (1000 mg/day) for 14 days. Ciprofloxacin appears to be safer with less risk for adverse effects. Rifaximin (1000 to 2000 mg/day) with or without concurrent use of ciprofloxacin or metronidazole may also be used for induction therapy. If patients respond to antibacterial therapy and have infrequent relapses (eg, 4 or fewer flare-ups in a 12-month period), they can be classified as having antibiotic-responsive pouchitis and treated with the same antibiotic used initially. If patients initially respond to antibiotics, but have frequent flare-ups requiring multiple courses of antibiotics, those patients may be treated as antibiotic-dependent pouchitis. These patients often require long-term antibiotic treatment to keep the disease in remission, either with a low-dose maintenance therapy or with pulse therapy. Patients on maintenance antibiotics who develop loss of clinical benefit after prolonged treatment, rotation of antibiotics such as metronidazole, ciprofloxacin, rifaximin, and tinidazole, may be attempted. For patients with antibiotic-dependent pouchitis, probiotic agents may be tried.

Chronic antibiotic-refractory pouchitis is a condition in which patients fail to respond to 2 to 4 weeks of single antibiotic therapy and is a common cause of pouch failure. In patients who have chronic antibiotic refractory pouchitis resistant to a routine single antibiotic, a combination of 2 antibiotics (ciprofloxacin with tinidazole, rifaximin, or metronidazole) can be administetered. Patients who do not respond to these antibiotic agents may be considered for other treatments with immunomodulators and biological agents. Before instituting antibiotics, the other causes of refractory disease including use of NSAIDs, *C. difficile,* cytomegalovirus or fungal infection, celiac disease, and other autoimmune disorders should be evaluated. Figure 18-1 summarizes the approach to the classification and management of pouchitis.

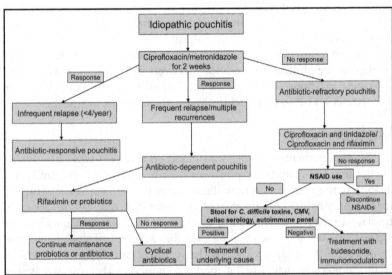

**Figure 18-1.** Classification and management of pouchitis.

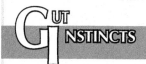

POUCHITIS

1. Pouchitis is the most frequent long-term complication of IPAA in patients with UC, with a cumulative prevalence of up to 50%.
2. Pouchitis can be classified based on the etiology into idiopathic pouchitis and secondary pouchitis.
3. *C. difficile*, cytomegalovirus, and NSAID-induced pouchitis are the common causes of secondary pouchitis.
4. Pouchitis can be classified based on patient response to antibiotics, as acute antibiotic-responsive entity, antibiotic-dependent, and chronic antibiotic-refractory pouchitis.
5. Antibiotic therapy is the cornerstone of treatment for acute antibiotic-responsive pouchitis with a good therapeutic response to ciprofloxacin or metronidazole in most patients. Antibiotic-dependent pouchitis is more challenging, and patients often require long-term maintenance therapy with antibiotics to keep disease in remission. Treatment of chronic antibiotic-refractory pouchitis is often difficult, and immunomodulators and biological agents often are required.

## Key References

1. Wu H, Shen B. Pouchitis and pouch dysfunction. *Med Clin North Am.* 2010;94:75-92.
2. Navaneethan U, Shen B. Secondary pouchitis: those with identifiable etiopathogenetic or triggering factors. *Am J Gastroenterol.* 2010;105:51-64.
3. Navaneethan U, Shen B. Pros and cons of antibiotic therapy for pouchitis. *Expert Rev Gastroenterol Hepatol.* 2009;3:547-559.
4. Pardi DS, D'Haens G, Shen B, Campbell S, Gionchetti P. Clinical guidelines for the management of pouchitis. *Inflamm Bowel Dis.* 2009;15:1424-1431.

# CHAPTER 19

# Diarrhea

Lynn Shapiro Connolly, MD and
Eric Esrailian, MD, MPH

Diarrhea often means different things to patients and providers. It is a term used to describe loose or watery stools, increased stool frequency (more than 3 bowel movements a day), or an excessive volume of stool (more than 200 g per day). People at the highest risk of developing diarrhea are immunocompromised persons, those exposed to contaminated food or water, travelers, and those in close contact with infants and children. Diarrhea can be either acute or chronic (more than 4 weeks in duration), and it is usually due to one of the following mechanisms: osmotic, secretory, malabsorption/maldigestion, or inflammatory/exudative.

## Initial Approach to the Patient With Diarrhea

A thorough clinical history is critical for developing a diagnostic strategy. The pattern and duration of diarrhea, stool characteristics, and the presence of fecal incontinence must be ascertained. Clinicians should ask specifically about occupational exposure; travel history; and associated symptoms including nausea, vomiting, abdominal pain, and constitutional symptoms. Certain clues in the history may point toward a specific diagnosis, including antibiotic exposure (*Clostridium difficile*), recent travel (*Giardia lamblia* or amebiasis), food consumption (*Escherichia coli*), bloody stool or fever (inflammatory, infectious, neoplastic), oil droplets in the stool (malabsorption), excessive flatus (lactose intolerance), weight loss (inflammatory bowel disease

Esrailian E. *Gut Instincts: A Clinician's Handbook of Digestive and Liver Diseases* (pp 129-136).
© 2012 Taylor & Francis Group

[IBD], malignancy), day care exposure (*Giardia, Cryptosporidium, Shigella*), pregnancy (*Listeriosis*), and abdominal surgery/resection (malabsorption). Recipients of anal intercourse are prone to gonorrhea proctitis, chlamydia, herpes simplex, syphilis, and *Entamoeba histolytica*.

The physical examination is a useful marker of both the severity and the etiology. For example, oral ulcers, arthritis, erythema nodosum, or pyoderma gangrenosum may indicate IBD. Dermatitis herpetiformis suggests celiac sprue. Lymphadenopathy suggests small bowel lymphoma, acquired immune deficiency syndrome, or malignancy. Edema, muscle atrophy, cheilosis, glossitis, and tetany suggest malabsorption. A digital rectal examination should always be performed to assess sphincter competence and the presence of blood, anal fissures, and fistulas.

## Acute Diarrhea

Acute diarrhea is defined as diarrhea lasting fewer than 3 or 4 weeks and is often from viruses, bacteria, food poisoning, or medications. A great majority of acute infectious gastroenteritis is probably viral as stool cultures in these patients have been positive in only 1.5% of cases. Rotavirus and norovirus should be considered when patients have been exposed to day care centers, nursing homes, or cruise ships. In immunocompromised patients, cytomegalovirus (CMV) and herpes simplex virus (HSV) must be ruled out.

Acute bloody diarrhea suggests bacterial colitis, IBD, ischemic colitis, or even radiation colitis if the history makes sense. The 4 most common bacterial enteropathogens in the United States are *Campylobacter*, nontyphoid *Salmonella*, Shiga-toxin producing *E. coli* including 0157:H7, and *Shigella*. Eighty percent of travelers' diarrhea is bacterial in origin, with *E. coli* the most common. Most bacterial diarrhea is secondary to food-borne transmission.

Parasites are a rare etiology for acute infectious diarrhea but should be ruled out in certain situations. Recent travel, exposure to day care centers, and public waterborne outbreaks point toward *Giardia* and *Cryptosporidium*. Immunocompromised patients are at increased risk for *Cryptosporidium, Isospora belli, Cyclospora*, and *Microsporidia*.

Food poisoning usually resolves within 1 to 2 days and, in addition to diarrhea, may present with upper gastrointestinal symptoms. Symptoms that begin within 6 hours of ingestion are often due to a preformed toxin from *Staphyloccocus aureus* (spoiled mayonnaise). *Bacillus cereus* (reheated fried rice) causes symptoms within 8 to 12 hours. If symptoms begin 8 to 16 hours after ingestion, *Clostridium perfringens* is suggested (spoiled meat).

Diarrhea is a common side effect of medications including chemotherapy agents, H2-antagonists, diuretics, nonsteroidal anti-inflammatory drugs (NSAIDs), and elixir medicines containing lactose or sorbitol. Antibiotic-induced diarrhea secondary to *C. difficile* is often associated with fever, crampy abdominal pain, dysentery, and leukocytosis. Serious complications include toxic megacolon and colonic perforation.

## EVALUATION

Because most acute diarrhea is mild and self-limited, extensive workup is often not necessary or cost effective. Indications for a diagnostic evaluation include duration longer than 48 hours, severe diarrhea with dehydration, dysentery, fever, or severe abdominal pain. Diarrhea in elderly, immunocompromised, or hospitalized patients should also be investigated.

Stool cultures are not routinely recommended in most cases of watery diarrhea because of low yield. Indications for stool cultures include severe diarrhea (more than 6 unformed bowel movements per day), more than 1-week duration, fever, dysentery, and a local outbreak. The standard stool culture often only tests for *Salmonella*, *Shigella*, and *Campylobacter*. In most cases of infectious diarrhea, a single stool sample is satisfactory. Special stool studies may be needed for *E. coli* 0157:H7, other Shiga-toxin *E. coli*, *Vibrio* bacteria, and *C. difficile*.

Fecal hemoccult and fecal leukocyte tests are often ordered, but the ability of these studies to predict the presence of inflammatory diarrhea has varied greatly. A fecal lactoferrin latex agglutination assay has a higher sensitivity and specificity in distinguishing infectious from inflammatory diarrhea, but the test is not widely available. Stool ova and parasite studies may be sent if the patient has the aforementioned risk factors.

Endoscopy is uncommonly indicated for the diagnosis of acute diarrhea, with few exceptions such as distinguishing IBD from infectious diarrhea, and for possible opportunistic infections, such as CMV in immunocompromised patients.

## TREATMENT

Supportive care with fluid and electrolyte repletion is the mainstay of treatment in acute diarrhea. Antimotility agents (loperamide or diphenoxylate) and bismuth subsalicylate may be used in patients without fever or dysentery. These antidiarrheals should be titrated to control diarrhea, but avoid constipation.

Antibiotics are usually not required in acute diarrhea. Indications for antibiotics include febrile dysentery that is not due to Shiga-toxin producing *E. coli*, moderate to severe cases of travelers' diarrhea, and in patients with certain culture-proven pathogenic bacteria. Specific antibiotic therapy should be tailored to the pathogen. Patients who are suspected to have enterohemorrhagic *E. coli* (including O157:H7) should not receive antibiotics given the possible increased risk of hemolytic uremic syndrome. Healthy patients with mild nontyphoid-producing *Salmonella* infection should also not receive antibiotics because they prolong the excretion of organisms.

# Chronic Diarrhea

The American Gastroenterological Association suggests that chronic diarrhea be defined as a decrease in fecal consistency lasting 4 or more weeks. In developing countries, the most common causes of chronic diarrhea are irritable bowel syndrome, IBD (including microscopic colitis), chronic infections, and malabsorption syndromes (including celiac disease and lactose intolerance). A specific diagnosis can usually be achieved in more than 90% of patients. The history can often differentiate between functional and organic etiologies. Indicators for a functional etiology include a longstanding duration, lack of significant weight loss, absence of nocturnal diarrhea, and straining with defecation.

## EVALUATION

All patients who present with chronic diarrhea should have a complete blood count, chemistry panel, total protein, albumin, celiac serologies, and thyroid studies. Stool cultures are not routinely recommended in immunocompetent patients but may be considered in high-risk individuals. Most patients require some form of endoscopic evaluation (with sigmoidoscopy or colonoscopy and upper endoscopy for the small bowel) with mucosal biopsies even if endoscopically normal. If an inflammatory or neoplastic process is suspected, the clinician should consider small bowel imaging to evaluate for Crohn's disease, chronic infections, intestinal lymphoma, and neuroendocrine tumors.

A 24-hour quantitative stool collection is often useful in the workup for chronic diarrhea. Patients need to consume 80 to 100 g of fat during the collection and freeze the specimen. A daily fecal output greater than 7 g indicates steatorrhea and more than 14 g is specific for pancreatic or biliary steatorrhea. A low fecal pH (<5.3) is characteristic of carbohydrate malabsorption.

The stool osmotic gap is equal to 290 − 2 x (stool Na + stool K). A gap greater than 125 mOsm/kg suggests pure osmotic diarrhea, while a gap less than 50 mOsm/kg suggests pure secretory diarrhea. The differential diagnosis for osmotic diarrhea includes carbohydrate malabsorption, magnesium-induced diarrhea, and laxative abuse. Secretory diarrhea may be from infection, stimulant laxatives, medications, intestinal surgery, fatty acid malabsorption, celiac sprue, small intestinal bacterial overgrowth, tumors, or bile acid diarrhea.

In patients with secretory diarrhea, selective testing for gastrin (Zollinger-Ellison syndrome), calcitonin (thyroid medullary carcinoma), vasoactive intestinal polypeptide (neuroendocrine tumor), quantitative immunoglobulins (common variable immunodeficiency), urine 5-hydroxy indole acetic acid (carcinoid), and urine vanillylmandelic acid and metanephrine (pheochromocytoma) may be performed. With osmotic diarrhea, breath testing may be useful in determining carbohydrate malabsorption and small intestinal bacterial overgrowth.

## TREATMENT

The underlying disease should be treated for chronic diarrhea. Empiric therapy is used in three situations: as an initial treatment before diagnostic testing, when a diagnosis cannot be made, and when a diagnosis has been made but either no treatment is available or the treatment fails. The mainstay of treatment includes antimotility agents (loperamide, diphenoxylate, octreotide, and even tincture of opium), bile acid sequestrants (cholestyramine), and fiber. Table 19-1 summarizes treatment options.

| TABLE 19-1 | NONANTIBIOTIC EMPIRIC TREATMENT OPTIONS FOR DIARRHEA | | |
|---|---|---|---|
| Treatment | Used for | Special Instructions | Warnings/Limitations |
| Fluid and electrolyte repletion | Dehydration from diarrhea | Can try mixing ½-tsp salt, ½-tsp baking soda and 4-tbsp sugar in 1 L of water | Gatorade, fruit juices, and soda are hyperosmolar and deficient in electrolytes and, thus, are suboptimal replacements for patients with significant dehydration. |
| Bland diet | Acute diarrhea | Can try BRAT diet (bananas, rice, applesauce, and toast) | Viral or bacterial enteropathogens often result in transient lactase deficiency. Caffeine increases cyclic adenosine monophosphate levels, thus promoting secretion of fluid and worsening diarrhea. |
| Antimotility drugs | Acute and chronic diarrhea | | Avoid empiric use in patients with fever or dysentery. |
| Loperamide (Imodium) | Preferred antimotility drug for diarrhea; unlike other opiates, it does not penetrate the nervous system and has no substantial potential for addiction | 1 to 2 mg PO everyday to QID on a scheduled basis. Titrate to number of stools per day. Max 16 mg/day. | May cause dizziness, drowsiness, tiredness, or constipation. |
| Diphenoxylate with atropine (Lomotil) | There is no major advantage over Imodium | 1 to 2 tabs PO BID to QID on a scheduled basis. Titrate to number stools per day. Max 8 tabs or 40 mL/day. | More central opiate effects and may produce anticholinergic side effects from atropine. |

(continued)

| TABLE 19-1 | NONANTIBIOTIC EMPIRIC TREATMENT OPTIONS FOR DIARRHEA (CONTINUED) | | |
|---|---|---|---|
| Treatment | Used for | Special Instructions | Warnings/Limitations |
| Tincture of opium | Often used for chronic diarrhea | Start: 2 drops BID. Titrate up slowly prn. | Can be addictive. May cause constipation, dizziness, drowsiness, tiredness, nausea, vomiting, and blurred vision. |
| Bismuth subsalicylate (Pepto-Bismol) | Traveler's diarrhea, norovirus diarrhea, and diarrhea where vomiting is a predominant symptom | 30 mL by mouth every hour as needed. Max 120 mL/ 24 hours | Usually well tolerated, but can cause black stools and tongue. Caution that Pepto-Bismol contains aspirin. |
| Probiotics (including Lactobacillus) | Travelers' diarrhea and antibiotic-associated diarrhea | Daily. Dose depends on route of administration. | May cause gas or bloating. |
| Octreotide acetate (Sandostatin) | Carcinoid tumors and other peptide-secreting tumors, dumping syndrome, chemotherapy-induced diarrhea, and short bowel syndrome | Start: 200 to 300 mcg/ day SC/IV div BID to QID x 2 weeks then individualize dose. Titrate to desired effect; doses >450 mcg/day rarely needed. | Need to administer it parentally (SC or IV). Expensive. May cause nausea, vomiting, abdominal pain, headache, fatigue, dizziness, and constipation. |
| Cholestyramine | Diarrhea caused from high fecal bile acids | 2 to 4 g PO BID to QID. Max 16 g/day. | May cause constipation, abdominal pain, flatulence, nausea, and vomiting. |

BID indicates twice daily; QID, 4 times a day; PO, given orally; SC, subcutaneous; IV, intravenous

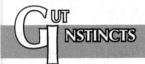
GUT INSTINCTS                                                        DIARRHEA

1. The medical history can be helpful in differentiating between functional and organic etiologies of diarrhea. Indicators for a functional etiology include a longstanding duration, lack of significant weight loss, and the absence of nocturnal symptoms.

2. Acute infectious diarrhea is usually mild and self-limited, so extensive workup is typically unnecessary. Most cases of acute infectious diarrhea are probably viral.

3. The 4 most common bacterial enteric pathogens in the United States are *Campylobacter*, non-typhoid *Salmonella*, Shiga-toxin producing *E. coli* including 0157:H7, and *Shigella*.

4. Patients who are suspected to have enterohemorrhagic *E. coli* (including 0157:H7) and healthy patients with mild nontyphoid producing *Salmonella* infection should not receive antibiotics.

5. Some common overlooked causes of diarrhea include diet (lactose intolerance, celiac disease), medications, inadvertent laxative use, irritable bowel syndrome, and occult infections.

## Key References

1. DuPont H. Bacterial diarrhea. *N Engl J Med*. 2009;361(16):1560-1569.
2. Fine K, Schiller L. AGA technical review on the evaluation and management of chronic diarrhea. *Gastroenterology*. 1999;116(6):1464-1486.
3. Headstrom PD, Surawicz CM. Chronic diarrhea. *Clin Gastroenterol Hepatol*. 2005;3(8):734-737.
4. Aranda-Michel J, Giannella R. Acute diarrhea: a practical review. *Am J Med*. 1999;106(6):680-676.

# CHAPTER 20

# CONSTIPATION

Lin Chang, MD

Chronic constipation is a common condition that consists of difficult, infrequent, or perceived incomplete defecation. The prevalence of chronic constipation ranges from 2% to 28%. Up to 63 million individuals in North America meet the diagnostic criteria for constipation. Epidemiologic studies demonstrate that the prevalence of constipation increases with age and is more common in women than men. A large disconnect exists between the perceptions of patients and health care providers regarding the defining symptoms of constipation. While health care providers generally rely on a frequency-based definition (ie, fewer than 3 bowel movements per week), patients perceive constipation as symptom based and often report that straining is their most bothersome symptom.

## Causes of Chronic Constipation

Chronic constipation is often characterized as being either primary or secondary (ie, due to an organic medical condition or use of a medication). Secondary causes of chronic constipation include structural lesions (eg, colon cancer, colonic strictures), endocrine and metabolic diseases (eg, diabetes, hypothyroidism), neurologic diseases (eg, Hirschsprung's disease, Parkinson's disease), myopathic conditions (eg, scleroderma, myotonic dystrophy), and other (eg, pregnancy, medications). The majority of the secondary causes may be excluded by

Esrailian E. *Gut Instincts: A Clinician's Handbook of Digestive and Liver Diseases* (pp 137-144).
© 2012 Taylor & Francis Group

| TABLE 20-1 | ROME III CRITERIA FOR FUNCTIONAL CONSTIPATION |
|---|---|

Symptoms must be present for the past 3 months with symptom onset at least 6 months prior to diagnosis. All 3 of the following criteria must be met:

1. Must include at least 2 of the following:
   - Straining during at least 25% of defecations
   - Lumpy or hard stools in at least 25% of defecations
   - Sensation of incomplete evacuation for at least 25% of defecations
   - Sensation of anorectal obstruction/blockage for at least 25% of defecations
   - Manual maneuvers to facilitate at least 25% of defecations (eg, digital evacuation, support of the pelvic floor)
   - Fewer than 3 defecations per week
2. Loose stools are rarely present without the use of laxatives
3. There are insufficient criteria for IBS

a thorough history and physical examination combined with limited laboratory studies. The primary pathophysiologic causes of chronic constipation (ie, functional constipation) can be divided into 3 main subtypes: normal transit, slow transit, and dyssynergic (or defecatory) dysfunction. In normal-transit constipation, the rate of stool passage through the colon and stool frequency are normal, but patients perceive they are constipated. In slow-transit constipation, passage of stool through the colon is slower than normal. Defecatory disorders, which include dyssynergic defecation, rectal prolapse, and rectocele, can also cause chronic constipation. In dyssynergic dysfunction, also referred to as pelvic floor dysfunction or anismus, there is ineffective coordination of the pelvic floor, abdominal, rectal, and anal sphincter musculature in the evacuation mechanism.

# Definition of Functional Constipation

Functional constipation is diagnosed using symptom-based criteria. The Rome III criteria are currently used to diagnose functional constipation (Table 20-1). It is important to differentiate functional constipation from irritable bowel syndrome (IBS) with constipation because the management approach may differ. IBS can be most easily distinguished from functional constipation by the presence of predominant abdominal pain associated with constipation. Patients cannot meet the diagnostic criteria for functional constipation if they meet diagnostic criteria for IBS.

# Diagnostic Evaluation of Chronic Constipation

Although differentiating constipation by subtype may help guide treatment decisions, an extensive diagnostic evaluation is not recommended in the absence of alarm features (eg, blood in the stool, unintentional weight loss, family history of colon cancer). Laboratory tests that may be useful include thyroid function tests, a complete blood count, serum electrolytes, serum calcium, and glucose levels. All average-risk patients older than age 50 should undergo routine colorectal cancer screening. In select patients, such as those with refractory symptoms, more specialized diagnostic testing may be considered, which includes colon transit studies, anorectal manometry with balloon expulsion testing, barium defecography, colon manometry, and pelvic floor magnetic resonance imaging (MRI).

# Slow Transit Constipation

Gut transit refers to the time taken for food or other material to pass through the gastrointestinal (GI) tract. The most commonly used technique to measure colonic transit in clinical practice is with radio-opaque markers. There are several ways to use this technique. Patients are given 1 capsule containing 24 radio-opaque markers, and an abdominal radiograph is obtained at day 5. A normal study is retention of less than 20% of markers. Another method involves having the patient take a capsule daily for 3 consecutive days and obtaining an abdominal radiograph on days 4 and 7. It is important that patients are instructed not to take any prokinetic or laxative agents during the course of the study because the test will likely not accurately reflect true colon transit time. Scintigraphy is another validated technique to measure GI transit and is frequently used to measure change in transit time in chronic constipation and IBS treatment trials. A newer technique is a wireless capsule that measures motility, pH, and temperature simultaneously.

Slow transit constipation typically occurs in young women and is often manifested by infrequent bowel movements and lack of urge to defecate. Delayed transit of radio-opaque markers through the colon usually suggests the presence of slow transit constipation; however, it can also be due to a defecatory disorder (see p. 140). When slowed transit is present, a defecatory disorder should be excluded by an anorectal manometry, rectal balloon expulsion test, and/or defecogram. A high-fiber diet can help improve stool passage in mild-moderate cases. Laxatives, chloride channel activator (ie, lubiprostone), and/or prokinetic agents (eg, the 5-$HT_4$ agonist prucalopride, which is currently only available in Europe) can provide relief of constipation symptoms that are refractory to fiber supplementation or in more moderate to severe cases.

# Dyssynergic Defecation

Constipation associated with anorectal dysfunction has been referred to as anismus, pelvic floor dyssynergia, obstructive defecation, paradoxical puborectalis contraction, pelvic outlet obstruction, and spastic pelvic floor syndrome. The term now recommended by experts is *dyssynergic defecation*. Failure of rectoanal coordination can be due to impaired rectal contraction, paradoxical anal contraction, and/or inadequate anal relaxation. Two-thirds of affected individuals acquire this condition in adulthood. Associated factors include excessive straining to evacuate hard stools, history of physical or sexual abuse, pregnancy, childbirth trauma, back injury, and structural abnormalities such as a rectocele or rectal intussusception. In about 40% of cases, there is no inciting cause.

Use of manual maneuvers and anal pain are suggestive of dyssynergic defecation. Digital rectal examination and anorectal manometry with balloon expulsion test can be helpful in diagnosing dyssynergic defecation. Digital rectal examination should be performed to assess anal sphincter tone at rest and during squeeze command and to exclude the presence of a stricture, mass, or blood. The presence of paradoxical pelvic floor contraction may be indicative of dyssynergic defecation, which can be assessed by asking the patient to bear down as if to defecate. The examiner should evaluate if the proper push and bear down technique is being performed (ie, the patient should be able to relax his or her external anal sphincter and puborectalis muscles with pelvic floor descent). The examiner should also place his or her left hand on the abdomen to determine if an appropriate abdominal wall contraction and push effort is made. If paradoxical pelvic floor contraction is present, particularly in a patient who is refractory to conventional constipation treatment, the patient should be referred for anorectal manometry and balloon expulsion test.

The presence of a dyssynergic anorectal manometric pattern during push command and an inability to expel a 50-mL water-filled rectal balloon are suggestive of dyssynergic defecation. Other tests that can help diagnose dyssynergic defecation include a delayed colon transit (eg, radio-opaque marker test) particularly in the rectosigmoid colon and an abnormal evacuation of barium paste on a defecogram. If there is evidence of dyssynergic defecation, the patient should be referred for anorectal biofeedback, which has been shown in controlled studies to be the most efficacious treatment for this condition.

## Management Options

In cases of secondary constipation, eliminating or switching the problematic medication or addressing the underlying condition may relieve the constipation. In patients in whom there is no secondary cause of constipation or alarm feature present, empiric treatment can be tried initially for functional constipation. Although fluid intake and exercise are often advocated to treat constipation, studies that demonstrate their significant benefit in the treatment of chronic constipation are lacking. Although the recommended daily fiber intake is 20 to 35 g, most Americans consume only 5 to 10 g daily. Patients who consume substantially less than the recommended minimum should be encouraged to increase their fiber intake by 5 g per day at 1-week intervals until the recommended intake is attained. Some patients may be particularly susceptible to significant bloating and cramps with sudden increases in fiber. A variety of pharmacologic treatment options exist for patients with chronic constipation. Treatment options should be selected based on the available evidence as well as individual patient preferences. Table 20-2 provides an overview of evidence-based therapies for chronic constipation.

## TABLE 20-2

## PHARMACOLOGIC TREATMENT FOR CHRONIC CONSTIPATION

| | Dosing | Efficacy | Safety | Comments |
|---|---|---|---|---|
| Bulking agents (psyllium) | Titrate up to 20 to 25 g per day | Improvements in stool frequency or consistency; no placebo-controlled trials using calcium polycarbophil or methylcellulose | Bloating and nausea. No drug interactions were demonstrated. | U.S. Food and Drug Administration (FDA) approved for use in occasional constipation. Suboptimal quality of studies. |
| Stool softeners | Docusate sodium/ calcium 100 mg PO QD to BID | Lack of high-quality studies | Diarrhea, abdominal cramps | FDA-approved for use in occasional constipation. Insufficient data to make a recommendation regarding efficacy. |
| Stimulant laxatives | Bisacodyl 5 to 15 mg PO QD<br><br>Senna 15 mg PO QD (maximum: 70 to 100 mg/day in BID dosing) | Majority of studies of poor methodological quality; recent placebo-controlled trial demonstrating efficacy of bisacodyl at a dose of 10 mg/day | Abdominal discomfort and cramps | FDA approved for use in occasional constipation |
| Osmotic laxatives | Lactulose 15 to 30 ml QD to BID PEG 3350 17 g/day | Good evidence demonstrated for use in occasional constipation and short-term constipation | Lactulose: Flatulence, intestinal cramps, and nausea PEG: Nausea, abdominal bloating, and cramping. Pregnancy category C. No drug interactions demonstrated for either drug. | FDA approved for use in occasional constipation |

(continued)

| TABLE 20-2 | PHARMACOLOGIC TREATMENT FOR CHRONIC CONSTIPATION (CONTINUED) | | | |
|---|---|---|---|---|
| | Dosing | Efficacy | Safety | Comments |
| Probiotics | *Lactobacillus casei* Shirota 65 mL/day | *Lactobacillus casei* Shirota improved self-reported constipation severity and stool consistency over placebo in patients with constipation | None reported with *Lactobacillus* in the study | Further data needed |
| 5-HT$_4$ agonists | Tegaserod 6 mg BID<br><br>Prucalopride 1 to 2 mg QD | Improved stool frequency, straining, and SBM compared with placebo | Diarrhea, headache<br><br>0.1% incidence of cardiovascular events with tegaserod versus 0.01% with placebo. Cardiovascular adverse events not demonstrated with prucalopride | Tegaserod is currently available only under emergency use IND for women aged <55 years with chronic idiopathic constipation or IBS-C in the United States.<br>Prucalopride is approved for use in Europe but not yet in the United States. |
| Type-2 chloride channel activator | Lubiprostone 24 mcg PO BID | Found to significantly increase SBM and reduce other constipation symptoms | Vomiting, nausea, and abdominal cramping; pregnancy category C | FDA approved for use in chronic constipation |

IBS-C indicates irritable bowel syndrome with constipation; PO, by mouth; BID, twice daily; QD, daily; SBM, spontaneous bowel movement; IND, investigational new drug; CC, chronic constipation; PEG, polyethylene glycol

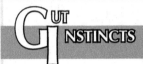

CONSTIPATION

1. Chronic constipation can be due to primary and secondary causes.

2. Constipation is characterized by a range of symptoms including hard stools, straining, sensation of incomplete evacuation, use of manual maneuvers, sensation of anorectal blockage, and decreased bowel movement frequency. The latter is reported in only about one-third of patients with self-reported constipation.

3. In the absence of alarm features, an extensive diagnostic evaluation is of low yield and is not indicated in patients who meet diagnostic symptom-based criteria for functional constipation.

4. Dyssynergic defecation should be suspected in patients with chronic constipation who report anal pain, use of manual maneuvers to facilitate stool evacuation, and/or prolonged straining and have failed conventional treatment.

5. Integrating an evidence-based and patient-centered approach can lead to successful management of chronic constipation.

## Key References

1. Brandt LJ, Prather CM, Quigley EMM, Schiller LR, Schoenfeld P, Talley NJ. Systematic review on the management of chronic constipation in North America. *Am J Gastroenterol.* 2005;(100 Suppl 1):S5-S22.

2. Lembo A, Camilleri M. Chronic constipation. *N Engl J Med.* 2003;349(14): 1360-1368.

3. Rao SC. Dyssynergic defecation and biofeedback therapy. *Gastroenterol Clin North Am.* 2008;37(3):569-586, viii.

# IRRITABLE BOWEL SYNDROME

Emeran A. Mayer, MD

## Definition and Epidemiology

Irritable bowel syndrome (IBS), characterized by chronically recurring abdominal pain or discomfort and altered bowel habits, is one of the most common syndromes seen by gastroenterologists and primary-care providers, with a worldwide prevalence of 10% to 15%. In the absence of detectable organic causes, IBS is currently referred to as a functional or symptom-based syndrome, which is defined by symptom criteria (see the ROME criteria in Table 21-1).

IBS is one of several functional gastrointestinal (GI) disorders (including functional dyspepsia), and these other functional disorders are frequent in IBS patients. Other pain disorders, such as fibromyalgia, chronic pelvic pain, and interstitial cystitis, are often comorbid in IBS patients. Psychological comorbidities are also common, primarily anxiety, somatization (presence of multiple somatic complaints), and symptom-related fears. These issues contribute to impairments in quality of life and excessive health care utilization associated with IBS.

Symptoms characteristic of IBS are common in population-based samples of healthy individuals. However, only 25% to 50% of individuals with such symptoms (typically those with more frequent or severe abdominal pain) seek medical care. Longitudinal studies suggest substantial fluctuations in symptoms over time. Symptoms can wax and wane, and transition to other GI symptom complexes (eg, functional dyspepsia) may occur over time.

Esrailian E. *Gut Instincts: A Clinician's Handbook of Digestive and Liver Diseases* (pp 145-154).
© 2012 Taylor & Francis Group

| TABLE 21-1 | ROME DIAGNOSTIC CRITERIA*<br>FOR IRRITABLE BOWEL SYNDROME |
|---|---|

Recurrent abdominal pain or discomfort at least 3 days/month in the past 3 months associated with 2 or more of the following:

1. Improvement with defecation.

2. Onset associated with a change in frequency of stool.

3. Onset associated with a change in form (appearance) of stool.

*Criteria fulfilled for the past 3 months with symptom onset at least 6 months prior to diagnosis.

Based on the predominant bowel habit, IBS has been subdivided into subgroups: IBS-M (mixed), IBS-D (diarrhea; more common in men), and IBS-C (constipation; more common in women), each group accounting for about one-third of all patients.

According to current diagnostic criteria, IBS has to be differentiated from functional abdominal pain syndrome (in IBS, abdominal pain symptoms have to be associated with alterations in bowel movements), from chronic functional constipation, and from chronic functional diarrhea (in IBS, pain/discomfort has to be associated with altered bowel habits).

Symptoms of IBS (or other related functional GI symptoms) frequently date back to childhood. The estimated prevalence of IBS in children is similar to that in adults. The female-to-male ratio is 2:1 in most population-based samples and is higher among those who seek health care. About 10% of adult patients develop IBS-like symptoms following bacterial or viral enteric infections. Risk factors for developing postinfectious IBS include female gender, a longer duration of gastroenteritis, and psychosocial factors (including a major life stress at the time of infection and high scores of somatization). Both initial presentations and exacerbations of IBS symptoms are often preceded by major psychological or physical (GI infection) stressors.

Given the sensitivity of IBS symptoms to stress and the responsiveness of symptoms in many individuals to therapies directed at the central nervous system, IBS is often described as a brain-gut disorder. Alterations in GI motility and possibly intestinal fluid handling may underlie bowel habit irregularities. These abnormalities may be mediated in part by dysregulation of the gut-based serotonin-signaling system and/or by altered autonomic nervous system regulation of the gut. Visceral hypersensitivity may contribute to abdominal pain and discomfort. Preliminary reports suggest contributions by alterations in the intestinal microflora, but a causative role in IBS symptoms remains to be established.

## Evaluation

According to current clinical guidelines, IBS can generally be diagnosed without additional testing (in particular, without colonoscopy) in patients who have symptoms meeting ROME criteria (see Table 21-1) and in the absence of "red flags." Red flags include rectal bleeding, anemia, weight loss, fever, family history of colon cancer, first symptom onset after age 50, or major symptom changes. Patients should be questioned regarding specifics of bowel habits and stool characteristics and, according to predominant bowel habits, can be subclassified into IBS with diarrhea (IBS-D), IBS with constipation (IBS-C), or mixed bowel habit (IBS-M). The differential diagnosis in ROME-positive IBS patients without red flags is small, but includes celiac disease, microscopic colitis, atypical Crohn's disease for IBS-D, and chronic constipation (without pain) for IBS-C. A relationship of symptoms to food intake, as well as possible "triggers" for onset of symptoms (eg, GI infection or significant stressors), should be assessed because they may guide treatment recommendations. In addition, attention is warranted to symptoms suggestive of other functional GI, somatic pain disorders, and psychological morbidities often associated with IBS.

Clinical experience suggests that accepting the patient's symptoms and distress as real, and not simply as a manifestation of excessive worrying and somatization, and providing the patient with a plausible model of his or her disease (brain-gut disorder) facilitates the establishment of a positive patient-doctor relationship. Physical examination may be normal, but frequently reveals tenderness in the left lower quadrant over an often palpable sigmoid colon. A rectal examination is warranted to exclude rectal pathology and abnormal anorectal sphincter function (eg, paradoxical pelvic floor contraction during a defecation attempt), which may contribute to constipation symptoms.

## Treatment

Patients with mild symptoms seen in primary-care settings typically get satisfactory relief of their symptoms from symptomatic treatment (usually aimed at normalizing bowel habits or decreasing abdominal pain) by a reassuring health care provider. However, the treatment of patients with more severe symptoms remains challenging. Only a small number of pharmacological and psychological treatments are supported by well-designed randomized controlled trials (RCTs) in patients with IBS.

## PHARMACOTHERAPY

Pharmacotherapy of IBS with currently available drugs is typically targeted to the management of individual symptoms, such as constipation, diarrhea, and abdominal pain (Table 21-2).

### Constipation

In clinical practice, osmotic laxatives are often useful in treating constipation, although these have not been studied in clinical trials specifically in patients with IBS. Fiber and other bulking agents have also been used as initial therapy for constipation. However, the frequent side effects (in particular, an increase in bloating) and inconsistent, largely negative results of trials of dietary fiber in the treatment of IBS have decreased the use of this approach. Nevertheless, such a baseline approach may benefit some patients. Newer drugs for constipation are being developed, based on the concept of stimulating intestinal secretion, which, in turn, will increase propulsive colonic activity. Lubiprostone (8 mcg bid) is the first such drug that has been approved by the US Food and Drug Administration (FDA) for IBS-C.

### Diarrhea

Although randomized trials for traditional antidiarrheal agents in IBS-D are lacking, clinical experience indicates that these agents are generally effective. Regular use of low doses (eg, loperamide 2 mg every morning after breakfast or twice daily) appears useful in treating otherwise uncontrollable diarrhea and may decrease patients' anxiety over uncontrollable urgency and fecal soiling. A drug studied specifically in patients with IBS-D is the $5-HT_3$ receptor, antagonist alosetron. In large randomized double-blind, placebo-controlled trials, alosetron (1 mg twice daily for 12 weeks) decreased stool frequency and bowel urgency, relieved abdominal pain and discomfort, and improved global IBS symptom scores and health-related quality of life. However, despite its effectiveness, the FDA has restricted the use of the drug due to rare, but serious, adverse effects occurring in both clinical trials and post-marketing studies, including complications from constipation and ischemic colitis. Therefore, alosetron is currently only indicated for women with severe IBS-D who have experienced chronic symptoms for at least 6 months and who have not responded to conventional therapies.

| TABLE 21-2 | MEDICATIONS USED IN THE TREATMENT OF IRRITABLE BOWEL SYNDROME* | | | | | | |
|---|---|---|---|---|---|---|---|

| Symptom and Medication | Initial Dose (mg/day) | Target Dose (mg/day) | Common or Serious Side Effects | Evidence C | Evidence IBS | FDA Approved C | FDA Approved IBS |
|---|---|---|---|---|---|---|---|
| *Constipation* | | | | | | | |
| Laxatives[1] | 17 g | 70 x (10³) | Diarrhea, bloating, cramping | ++ | - | - | - |
| Polyethylene glycol 3350 (Miralax) | | 20 to 40 x 10³ | Diarrhea, bloating, cramping | + | - | - | - |
| Lactulose (Kristalose) | | | | ++ | | | |
| Secretory stimulators | 10 to 20 g | | Nausea, diarrhea, headache, abdominal pain/discomfort | + | ++ | Yes | Yes |
| Lubiprostone[2] (Amitizia, Succampo) | | 8 mcg BID | | ++ + | | | |
| *Diarrhea* | | | | *D* | *IBS* | *D* | *IBS* |
| Loperamide (Imodium) | 2 | 2 to 8 | Constipation | ++ | - | Yes | No |
| Alosetron (Lotronex)[3] | | 0.5 mg BID | Constipation, ischemic colitis (rare) | + | ++ | No | Yes[4] |

(continued)

| Table 21-2 | Medications Used in the Treatment of Irritable Bowel Syndrome* (continued) | | | | | | |
|---|---|---|---|---|---|---|---|
| **Symptom and Medication** | **Initial Dose (mg/day)** | **Target Dose (mg/day)** | **Common or Serious Side Effects** | **Evidence** | | **FDA Approved** | |
| | | | | B | IBS | B | IBS |
| *Bloating* | | | | | | | |
| Antibiotics | | | | | | | |
| Rifaxin (Xifaxin) | | 400 TID | Abdominal pain, diarrhea, bad taste | - | + | No | No |
| Probiotics[4] | | | | | | | |
| *Bifidobacterium infantis* 35624 (Align) | | 4 QD | N/A | + | + | No | No |
| *Bifidobacterium lactis* DN 173 010 (Activia yogurt) | | 2 pods/d | N/A | + | + | No | No |
| *Pain* | | | | P | IBS | P | IBS |
| Antidepressants | | | | | | | |
| • TCAs[5] | | | Dry mouth, dizziness, weight gain | | | | |
| • Amitryptline (Elavil,) | 10 QHS | 10 to 100 QHS | | ++ | + | No | No |
| • Desipramine (Norpramine) | 10 QHS | 10 to 100 QHS | | ++ | + | No | No |

*(continued)*

**TABLE 21-2** | **MEDICATIONS USED IN THE TREATMENT OF IRRITABLE BOWEL SYNDROME* (CONTINUED)**

| Symptom and Medication | Initial Dose (mg/day) | Target Dose (mg/day) | Common or Serious Side Effects | Evidence | | FDA Approved | |
|---|---|---|---|---|---|---|---|
| | | | | P | IBS | P | IBS |
| *Pain* | | | | | | | |
| SSRI | | | | | | | |
| • Paroxetine CR (Paxil CR) | | 10 to 60 | Sexual dysfunction, headache, nausea, sedation, insomnia, sweating, withdrawal symptoms | - | + | No | No |
| • Escitalopram oxalate (Lexapro) | | 5 to 20 | | + | + | No | No |
| | | 20 to 40 | Somnolence, dizziness, headaches, insomnia | + | - | No | No |

* This list is not exhaustive, but includes major medications for which there is evidence from well-designed clinical trials for effectiveness for global irritable bowel syndrome symptoms or for individual symptoms (eg, constipation, diarrhea, abdominal pain/discomfort)

+ some evidence from at least one controlled trial; ++ moderate evidence from several controlled trials or from meta-analysis of such trials; +++ strong evidence from well-designed, controlled clinical trials.

C indicates constipation; D, diarrhea; B, bloating; P, pain (somatic or abdominal)

1 A wide range of osmotic and irritant laxatives, including fiber products are available over the counter (OTC).

2 Lubiprostone is approved by the US Food and Drug Administration (FDA) for the treatment of chronic constipation.

3 Lotronex use is restricted for women with severe IBS-D, unresponsive to other medications, due to side effects.

4 A wide range of probiotics are available OTC and are not listed. Shown is a probiotic for which a beneficial effect for IBS symptoms has been demonstrated in high-quality randomized controlled trials.

5 A wide range of different tricyclic antidepressants with varying side effects and side-effect profiles are available. Two commonly prescribed TCAs are listed.

# Abdominal Pain

## ANTISPASMODIC AGENTS

Antispasmodic agents (eg, hyoscyamine or mebeverine) have commonly been used for pain. However, data are lacking from high-quality RCTs to support their effectiveness in reducing pain or global symptoms. Empirical evidence suggests that antispasmodics may be useful in patients in whom a contracted, tender sigmoid colon is palpable.

## CENTRALLY ACTING DRUGS

Tricyclic antidepressant (TCA) medications are commonly used for IBS symptoms, often in low doses (eg, amitriptyline 10 to 75 mg). Hypothesized mediators of their effects include antihyperalgesia, improvement in sleep, normalization of GI transit, and, when used at higher doses (>100 mg QHS), treatment of comorbid depression and anxiety. Despite their frequent use in practice, evidence to support the efficacy of TCAs in IBS patients is inconsistent. In the largest randomized placebo-controlled trial to date, treatment with desipramine (escalating dose from 50 to 150 mg) was not superior to placebo in intention-to-treat analyses. Effects of TCAs on somatic pain sensitivity and sleep suggest that they may have particular benefit in IBS patients with widespread somatic pain or poor sleep, although this has not been explicitly studied.

Several small RCTs suggest that selective serotonin reuptake inhibitors (SSRIs) may have beneficial effects in IBS patients, most commonly on measures of general well being and, in some studies, on abdominal pain. However, it remains to be determined if this benefit was secondary to improvement in depression or anxiety. Although serotonin and norepinephrine reuptake inhibitors (SNRIs) duloxetine and venlafaxine have been shown to be effective in reducing pain in other chronic pain conditions, including fibromyalgia, data are lacking from RCTs to guide their role in IBS.

Despite a high prevalence of comorbid anxiety in patients with IBS, benzodiazepines are generally not recommended for chronic therapy due to the risk of habituation and potential for dependency. However, limited treatment of patients with high comorbid anxiety with low-dose clonazepam (0.25 mg twice daily) may be beneficial in selected patients.

## COGNITIVE BEHAVIORAL THERAPY

Cognitive behavioral therapy (CBT) is the best-studied psychological treatment for IBS. Cognitive techniques (whether administered in group or individual format over 4 to 15 sessions) are aimed at changing catastrophic or maladaptive thinking patterns underlying the perception of somatic symptoms. Gut-directed hypnosis (containing suggestions aimed at improving gut function) is a well-studied treatment involving relaxation, change in belief systems, and self-management. Some RCTs show support for its therapeutic value in reducing somatic symptoms. The magnitude of improvement that has been reported in clinical trials with psychological treatments appears similar to or greater than that reported with medications studied specifically for bowel symptoms in IBS, and the estimated number needed to treat (NNT) with CBT or hypnotherapy for one patient to achieve improvement was estimated to be 2.

# Summary and Recommendations

Based on the generally accepted model of altered brain-gut interactions in IBS, treatment approaches aimed at the gut (prokinetics, secretagogues, antidiarrheals, microflora-altering strategies) as well as centrally-targeted therapies, or combinations of the 2 approaches, may be effective in certain patients. A good patient-physician relationship and the communication of a rational disease model to the patient are essential for positive treatment outcomes. Once a positive diagnosis is made based on symptom criteria and red flags have been excluded, the diagnostic yield from additional diagnostic tests is minimal and should be avoided. Baseline therapies should include lifestyle recommendations, laxatives, or antidiarrheals (for altered bowel habits), as well as low-dose TCAs (for abdominal pain). In unresponsive patients, additional drugs, such as lubiprostone (for constipation) or alosetron (for refractory diarrhea), should be considered. In pain-predominant patients who have not responded to low-dose TCAs, nonselective reuptake inhibitors such as venlafaxine, duloxetine, or milnacipram may be considered. A cognitive behavioral approach should be used whenever available and acceptable to the patient.

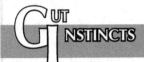

## IRRITABLE BOWEL SYNDROME

1. In the great majority of patients, the diagnosis of IBS can be made based on the ROME criteria and the absence of red flags. Additional diagnostic tests rarely lead to a change in the initial diagnosis and should be avoided.

2. The majority of IBS patients improve as a consequence of a good doctor-patient relationship, which includes the communication of a plausible brain-gut model and simple recommendations for lifestyle changes.

3. IBS patients are more prone to drug side effects and require starting with the lowest doses of medications, with slow titration to individual doses. Detailed explanations of drug mechanism and side effects reduce side effects.

4. Baseline therapies include probiotics, low-dose tricyclic antidepressants and, sometimes, antispasmodics and antidiarrheals.

5. Second-line therapies include novel secretagogues and nonselective reuptake inhibitors.

## Key References

1. Mayer EA. Clinical perspectives: irritable bowel syndrome. *N Engl J Med.* 2008;358(16):1692-1699.
2. Drossman DA. The functional gastrointestinal disorders and the Rome III process. *Gastroenterol.* 2006;130(5):1377-1390.
3. Drossman DA, Camilleri M, Mayer EA, Whitehead WE. AGA technical review on irritable bowel syndrome. *Gastroenterol.* 2002;123(6):2108-2131.

*Acknowledgments.* The author thanks Teresa Olivas and Cathy Liu for invaluable assistance in preparing the manuscript.

# SMALL INTESTINAL BACTERIAL OVERGROWTH

The digestive tract is host to a large diversity of bacterial flora. Each area has its own unique type and number of flora. Having the slowest transit time, the colon is the largest reservoir of bacteria in the human body. There is an estimated $10^{11}$ bacteria for every milliliter of colon contents. The human small bowel has a series of principles that prevent the accumulation of bacteria in this location. When any of these mechanisms fail, the small intestine can readily accumulate bacteria from the colon, and this leads to small intestinal bacterial overgrowth (SIBO). In this chapter, the principles of SIBO will be discussed in addition to treatment options.

## Definition

SIBO is defined as an excess of bacteria in the small intestine. As stated above, the small intestine contains few bacteria. In fact, some studies suggest that the upper small intestine is virtually sterile. The difficulty with this definition is that it can have many meanings. For example, in subjects with antrectomy and vagotomy, the lack of acid can lead to oral flora colonizing the upper small bowel. In other situations, such as distal ileal obstruction, the excessive flora is from the colon leading to a coliform SIBO. These 2 types of SIBO would have differing clinical implications. Most investigators refer to SIBO in the setting of coliform overgrowth.

Esrailian E. *Gut Instincts: A Clinician's Handbook of Digestive and Liver Diseases* (pp 155-160).
© 2012 Taylor & Francis Group

| TABLE 22-1 | STRENGTHS AND WEAKNESSES OF VARIOUS SUBSTRATES FOR BREATH TEST | |
| --- | --- | --- |
| Type of Substrate for Breath Test | Substrate | Detection of SIBO |
| Absorbable substrates | Glucose; sucrose | Rapid absorption by host gut, which makes substrate available over a limited portion of the gut.<br><br>A positive breath test is more likely to indicate SIBO because substrate should not reach colon.<br><br>High false-negative rate because much of the small bowel is not exposed to the substrate. |
| Low absorption substrates | Lactulose; xylose | Poor absorption makes substrate available.<br><br>Test for SIBO over the entire small bowel.<br><br>Rapid transit can mimic SIBO on this test and, therefore, these substrates have the potential for a high false-positive rate. |

Even coliform SIBO suffers from challenges in how it is defined in a given patient. Some state that culture of the small bowel is the gold standard for identifying SIBO. However, culture cannot be considered the gold standard because most gut organisms cannot be grown in culture and the ideal location for culture would be the distal small bowel, which cannot be easily accessed. In addition, tradition has stated that bacterial counts in excess of $10^5$ cfu/mL are consistent with SIBO. However, this value was obtained through studies of Billroth II and other subjects with severely altered anatomy. This value cannot be extrapolated to other disease states with intact bowel such as irritable bowel syndrome (IBS) or inflammatory bowel disease (IBD).

An alternative to culture is the use of breath testing. There are a number of substrates that can be used for breath testing. The most commonly used substrates in breath testing for SIBO are lactulose, glucose, and sucrose. The strengths and weaknesses of each of these substrates are summarized in Table 22-1. At this time, lactulose breath testing is the most common. Some investigators argue that the breath test for diagnosing SIBO is unreliable. However, because small bowel culture is not an adequate gold standard, there is no way to reliably determine the validity of breath testing. As seen in Table 22-1, the definitions of SIBO vary based on breath testing. The most commonly used definition of SIBO using the lactulose breath test was a rise of 20 ppm in hydrogen by 90 minutes after lactulose administration. Based on the lack of better tests, the breath test is likely to continue to be used as the best test for diagnosing SIBO.

# Pathophysiology and Risk Factors

The mechanisms that control bacterial populations and levels in the small bowel are complex and poorly understood, but some mechanisms that protect against the development of SIBO have been identified. The first of these is failure of the gastric acid barrier. Several studies have shown that inhibition of gastric acid secretion using omeprazole results in bacterial overgrowth and altered bowel function. In addition, pancreatic insufficiency due to chronic pancreatitis and cirrhosis have both been linked to SIBO, indicating that pancreatic and biliary secretions also play a role in controlling bacterial populations in the intestine. The ileocecal valve has been shown to play a role in preventing small bowel contamination, and ileal dysfunction has been linked to SIBO in patients with Crohn's disease. Studies of patients with immunodeficiency disorders have also demonstrated that mucosal immunity is also important in the prevention of SIBO. In addition, SIBO sometimes develops as a result of structural causes, such as blind intestinal loops or other iatrogenic surgically altered anatomy.

However, SIBO also occurs in a variety of conditions that are not associated with gross structural abnormalities, such as IBS. Subjects with IBS are more likely to have an abnormal breath test than controls, suggesting the presence of SIBO, and aspirates of jejunal fluid from IBS subjects exhibit a greater number of coliform bacteria than healthy controls. Alterations of gut motility have also been linked to SIBO, and a growing body of evidence suggests that this may contribute to the development of SIBO in IBS patients. Phase III of interdigestive motility, 1 of 3 components of normal fasting motility, is a high amplitude multiphasic motor event that cleanses debris from the small intestine after a meal, on a cycle of approximately 90 minutes. Patients with SIBO who did not have any structural abnormalities of the gut have been shown to exhibit reduced or absent Phase III events.

Lastly, an important group of organisms that colonize the gut are the methanogenic bacteria. This distinct group grows primarily under anaerobic conditions and produces methane ($CH_4$) as a byproduct of fermentation. Intestinal methane production has been linked to diseases

| TABLE 22-2 | GASES ON BREATH TESTING AND THEIR MEANING | |
|---|---|---|
| Type of Gas | Features | Clinical Association |
| Hydrogen ($H_2$) | Produced by large number of bacteria in the gut through fermentation<br><br>Rise of 20 ppm by 90 minutes after lactulose is considered by most to be a positive test for SIBO | Positive test with this gas often associated with diarrhea (although not believed to be cause and effect) |
| Methane ($CH_4$) | Produced by archaebacteria (most commonly *Methanobrevibacter smithii*)<br><br>Produced by using environmental hydrogen in intestine<br><br>Methane is rated as present or absent on breath testing (if >3 ppm) | Implicated in constipation<br><br>Methane gas has been shown to slow intestinal transit |
| Hydrogen sulfide ($H_2S$) | Produced by sulfate-reducing bacteria<br><br>Produced by using environmental hydrogen in intestine | Could be associated with a flat-line breath test<br><br>Because not measured, not yet associated with any clinical association |
| Carbon dioxide ($CO_2$) | Produced by bacteria, but cannot be discriminated from human metabolism<br><br>Used in breath testing to validate quality of breath sampling (alveolar $CO_2$ is fixed in concentration) | Could be associated with a flat-line breath test |

such as constipation-predominant IBS (C-IBS), diverticulosis, and other constipation disorders. In addition, the amount of methane produced is related to the degree of constipation, as measured by Bristol Stool Score and frequency of bowel movements. Table 22-2 describes gases detected on breath testing and their meaning.

## Treatment Options

Antibiotic therapy has traditionally been used to treat SIBO and specifically, has been successfully used to treat SIBO in patients suffering from functional bowel disease such as IBS. The first antibiotic used in a controlled trial to treat IBS on the basis of bacterial overgrowth was neomycin, which was found not only to result in significant improvement in IBS symptoms, but resulted in an average 75% improvement in IBS if lactulose breath tests were normalized, suggesting that eradication of SIBO was necessary and responsible for the improvement in IBS symptoms. However, the overall efficacy of the neomycin was low, as only 25% of breath tests were normalized after treatment with this antibiotic, and in those patients who did respond, when symptoms relapsed, 75% failed to respond to a second course of treatment, suggesting the development of clinical resistance to neomycin. Neomycin also does not have a favorable side-effect profile. Other antibiotics, such as doxycycline and ampicillin, were also subject to the same resistance issues. Subsequent studies have utilized rifaximin, which is a nonabsorbable broad-spectrum antibiotic with a low resistance profile. Rifaximin was initially found to have an efficacy of 70% in treating SIBO, and 3 subsequent randomized controlled trials demonstrated that rifaximin was successful in treating IBS patients on a SIBO basis. Significantly, patients treated with rifaximin remained improved for a full 10 weeks after cessation of antibiotic therapy, suggesting that the clinical resistance seen with neomycin did not occur with rifaximin. Thus, antibiotic-based therapies using rifaximin may be successful in treating SIBO associated with other functional bowel disorders in addition to IBS. Doses of rifaximin 400 to 550 mg, 3 times daily for 10 to 14 days, have been studied as an initial treatment, and additional data are still pending.

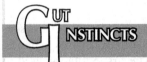

## BACTERIAL OVERGROWTH

1. SIBO may occur in a variety of conditions that are not associated with gross structural abnormalities, such as IBS.
2. There are no perfect diagnostic tests for SIBO.
3. Intestinal methane production has been linked to diseases such as C-IBS, diverticulosis, and other constipation disorders.
4. Rifaximin has been successfully used in treating some IBS patients on a SIBO basis.
5. Rifaximin doses of 400 to 550 mg, 3 times daily for 10 to 14 days, may be an effective initial treatment for SIBO.

## Key References

1. Khoshini R, Dai SC, Lezcano S, Pimentel M. A systematic review of diagnostic tests for small intestinal bacterial overgrowth. *Dig Dis Sci*. 2008;53(6): 1443-1454.
2. Ford AC, Spiegel BM, Talley NJ, Moayyedi P. Small intestinal bacterial overgrowth in irritable bowel syndrome: systematic review and meta-analysis. *Clin Gastroenterol Hepatol*. 2009;7(12):1279-1286.
3. Pimentel M, Park S, Mirocha J, Kane SV, Kong Y. The effect of a nonabsorbed oral antibiotic (rifaximin) on the symptoms of irritable bowel syndrome: a randomized trial. *Ann Intern Med*. 2006;145(8):557-563.

# CHAPTER 23

# LOWER GASTROINTESTINAL BLEEDING

Kunut Kijsirichareanchai, MD and
Rome Jutabha, MD

Lower gastrointestinal bleeding (LGIB) is generally referred to as blood loss emanating from the colorectal region of the digestive tract. Patients with LGIB most commonly present with hematochezia (bright red blood per rectum) or maroon-colored stools (coagulated blood/clots). Melena (black tarry stool) usually signifies upper gastrointestinal bleeding (UGIB), but can also occur in patients with LGIB if the bleeding originates from the cecum or right colon in the setting of slow colonic transit. Patients with severe LGIB, as evidenced by acute signs (eg, anemia, tachycardia, postural hypotension), or symptoms of hypovolemia (eg, dizziness, lightheadedness, presyncope) warrant an urgent evaluation and expedited resuscitation to avoid serious morbidity and mortality.

## Differential Diagnosis

### UPPER GASTROINTESTINAL BLEEDING

Approximately 10% of patients presenting with hematochezia actually have brisk UGIB with rapid transit of blood resulting in bright blood per rectum. Therefore, it is important to distinguish between LGIB and brisk UGIB because the patient prognoses, diagnostic tests, treatment options, and outcomes are quite different between the 2 conditions.

Esrailian E. *Gut Instincts: A Clinician's Handbook of Digestive and Liver Diseases* (pp 161-166).

## ANORECTAL LESIONS

A multitude of anorectal lesions can contribute to acute LGIB in patients who usually present with hematochezia. These anorectal lesions include internal hemorrhoids, anal fissures, ulcerative proctitis, radiation proctitis, rectal mass lesions (eg, polyps or carcinoma), and solitary rectal ulcer syndrome. Bleeding from these anorectal lesions is usually self-limited, is usually less severe as compared to colonic lesions, and can often be treated on an outpatient basis.

## DIVERTICULAR DISEASE

Colonic diverticulosis is the most common cause of LGIB in adults older than age 40, with the highest prevalence in patients older than 85 years. Diverticular bleeding can be brisk and life threatening due to its arterial origin of vasa recta, and it is usually painless. Diverticula can be found throughout the large intestine with the predominance in the left-side colon. It is noteworthy that the majority of diverticular bleeding emanates from the right side of the colon, whereas diverticulitis tends to occur in the left colon. Approximately 70% to 80% of diverticular bleeding is self-limited, but the rebleeding rate may be as high as 25%.

## ISCHEMIC COLITIS

Ischemic colitis is a relatively common (6% to 18%) and clinically important cause of LGIB especially in older patients who have cardiac risk factors that predispose to impaired blood flow to the colon, such as atherosclerotic vascular disease, congestive heart failure, cardiac arrhythmias, hypotensive state, or sepsis. Ischemic colitis usually presents as bloody diarrhea, often associated with cramping, in elderly patients who have one or more of the above predisposing risk factors. Cocaine and alpha-adrenergic medications have been associated with ischemic colitis in young patients without any cardiac risk factors. Bleeding from ischemic colitis is usually self-limited, and treatment includes intravenous (IV) fluids to restore colonic blood flow and prevent transmural injury (toxic megacolon).

## ANGIODYSPLASIA

Angiodysplasia, vascular ectasia, angiomata, and arterial venous malformation (AVM) are terms used to describe small (1 to 3 mm), capillary-like, dilated submucosal blood vessels that are commonly found in the ascending colon and cecum but can also be found anywhere throughout the digestive tract. Small bowel angiodysplasia is also a major cause of obscure gastrointestinal bleeding (GIB) and unexplained anemia in the adult population with an increased prevalence associated with older age. Colonic angiodysplasia is a major cause of LGIB, although recent studies have reported AVM-related LGIB as low as 1% in some large series.

## COLONIC INFLAMMATION/ULCERATION

Mucosal inflammation and ulceration due to acute or chronic colitis can present as severe lower GIB. The various causes of colitis-related LGI bleeding include infectious colitis (such as *Salmonella, Shigella, Campylobacter,* enteroinvasive *Escherichia coli, Cytomegalovirus*), drug-induced (eg, clindamycin-related *Clostridium difficile* colitis), vasculitis, ischemic colitis, inflammatory bowel diseases, and radiation-related colitis/proctitis.

## COLONIC MASS LESIONS

Benign polyps (hyperplastic, juvenile), neoplastic polyps (adenomas), or malignant mass lesions (adenocarcinoma) are important lesions to exclude for patients with hematochezia. Bleeding from mass lesions typically arises from mucosal ulceration eroding into an underlying blood vessel or auto-amputation of a pedunculated polyp at the stalk base. Colon polyps and colorectal cancer contribute to approximately 10% of LGIB cases.

## POSTPOLYPECTOMY-INDUCED ULCER BLEEDING

Routine colon cancer screening has led to an increase in colon polyp detection, as well as an increasing number of cases of delayed bleeding due to postpolypectomy-induced ulcers. Bleeding usually occurs within 1 to 2 weeks following polypectomy of large pedunculated polyps or large sessile polyps that require saline-assisted or piecemeal polypectomy. Patients who have an underlying coagulopathy, thrombocytopenia, or platelet dysfunction are at increased risk of developing postpolypectomy bleeding. Therefore, anticoagulation (warfarin [Coumadin], heparin) and anti-platelet (aspirin, nonsteroidal anti-inflammatory drugs [NSAIDs], clopidogrel) therapy should be withheld approximately 7 days following snare removal of large polyps if possible.

## SMALL BOWEL SOURCES

Small bowel bleeding accounts for approximately 10% of all GIB and can be mistaken for either LGIB or UGIB. Causes of small bowel bleeding include angiodysplasia, tumors (eg, lymphoma, carcinoid, polyps), Crohn's disease, NSAID-induced erosions and ulcers, and Meckel's diverticulum (in patients younger than 40 years old). The length (~21 feet) of the small intestine has made the diagnosis and treatment of small bowel pathology quite challenging. New capsule endoscopy devices and deep enteroscopy equipment are now available to evaluate and treat bleeding lesions within the small bowel.

## Initial Management

The initial management is similar to UGIB (see Chapter 9). Prompt evaluation and aggressive volume resuscitation are required for patients with hemodynamic instability or who have evidence of ongoing severe bleeding. Such patients should have 2 large-bore IV catheters for crystalloid solution and/or blood product transfusions as clinically indicated. Intensive level of care is highly recommended for close observation and monitoring of rebleeding, particularly within the first 24 to 48 hours after initial presentation.

## Diagnostic Approaches

A detailed history and physical examination including nasogastric tube lavage and digital rectal examination are important to assess the severity and possible sources of bleeding, but they often do not establish a definite diagnosis. Anoscopy can be performed at bedside to evaluate for suspected anorectal lesions. Colonoscopy is the initial diagnostic and therapeutic procedure of choice in patients with LGIB. If colonoscopy is nondiagnostic, upper endoscopy should be considered for patients with hematochezia and hemodynamic instability to exclude massive UGIB as the cause of rectal bleeding. Radionuclide scan (tagged red blood cell scan) may be useful to localize the bleeding region that might then be treated with angiography with embolizaiton. Bleeding patients with negative upper endoscopy and colonoscopy should undergo capsule endoscopy to identify possible small intestinal involvement. Positive findings from capsule endoscopy will warrant a need for deep enteroscopy (eg, push enteroscopy, single-balloon enterosocopy, double-balloon enteroscopy, spiral enteroscopy). Surgery (with or without concomitant intraoperative enteroscopy) might be required in some cases of refractory bleeding.

## Definitive Management

Most LGIB resolves spontaneously without any intervention or treatment. Many endoscopic treatment modalities are available to treat LGIB depending on the location and cause of the bleeding. These treatments include injection therapy (epinephrine, sclerosing agents), bipolar electrocoagulation (Gold probe, Bicap probe), argon plasma coagulation (APC), and hemoclips. Surgery usually is reserved for patients with recurrent or refractory bleeding who have failed or are not amenable to endoscopic or radiographic treatments. Figure 23-1 summarizes these diagnostic and management approaches.

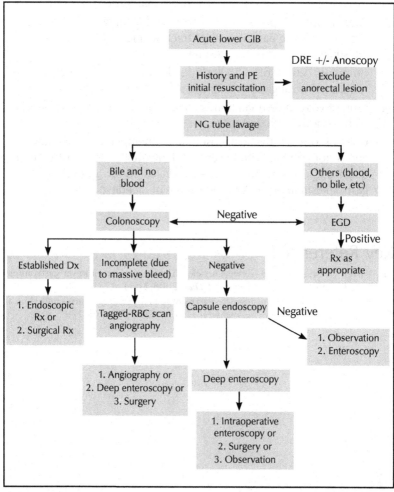

**Figure 23-1.** Lower gastrointestinal bleeding management algorithm. GI indicates gastrointestinal; PE, physical examination; DRE, digital rectal examination; NG, nasogastric; EGD, esophagogastroduodenoscopy; Dx, diagnosis; Rx, treatment; RBC, red blood cell.

# GUT INSTINCTS  LOWER GASTROINTESTINAL BLEEDING

1. LGIB refers to bleeding emanating from the colon or rectum that usually presents with hematochezia or maroon-colored stools.
2. Patients with suspected LGIB can have bleeding arising from any region along the gastrointestinal tract, including the upper gastrointestinal tract and small intestine.
3. Common causes of LGIB include diverticulosis, internal hemorrhoids, colitis, angiodysplasia, mass lesions, and ulcers.
4. Prompt volume resuscitation is critical for all patients who present with hemodynamic instability.
5. Colonoscopy is the diagnostic and therapeutic procedure of choice for patients with lower GIB. However, patients with a nondiagnostic colonoscopy should be evaluated for a possible upper gastrointestinal or small bowel source of bleeding.

## Key References
1. Farrell JJ, Friedman LS. Review article: the management of lower gastrointestinal bleeding. *Aliment Pharmacol Ther.* 2005;21(11):1281-1298.
2. Rockey DC. Occult and obscure gastrointestinal bleeding: causes and clinical management. *Nat Rev Gastroenterol Hepatol.* 2010;7(5):265-279.

# CHAPTER 24

# COLORECTAL CANCER AND SCREENING

Saeed Sadeghi, MD

Despite advances in understanding the epidemiology of colorectal cancer (CRC), as well as advances in chemoprevention and surveillance modalities, it remains the third most common cause of malignancy in both men and women, and the second leading cause of cancer death in the United States. Approximately 72% of CRC arise in the colon. The remaining 28% are below the peritoneal reflection (15 cm above the anal verge) and are considered to be rectal cancers.

Most CRC is sporadic. However, hereditary risk factors including a positive family history, familial adenomatous polyposis (FAP), and hereditary nonpolyposis CRC (HNPCC) are associated with an increased lifetime risk of CRC. In addition, underlying inflammatory bowel disease can further increase the CRC risk. Other risk factors include obesity, alcohol and red meat consumption, smoking history, and diabetes. While controlled studies have suggested a role for chemoprevention using calcium, nonsteroidal anti-inflammatory drugs (NSAIDs), and 3-hydroxy-3-methylglutaryl-coenzyme A (HMG-CoA) reductase inhibitors, the use of such agents is not a substitute for a comprehensive screening program.

## Screening

As part of the annual physical examination, digital rectal examination has the ability to detect low rectal lesions up to 7 cm from the

Esrailian E. *Gut Instincts: A Clinician's Handbook of Digestive and Liver Diseases* (pp 167-172).

anal verge. A fecal occult blood testing (FOBT), either guaiac-based or the fecal immunohistochemical test (FIT), should also be performed as part of the annual physical examination. Although FOBT has been routinely used as a screening tool, the test fails to identify the majority of CRC because patients are usually not bleeding at the time of the test. Despite this reality, randomized controlled trials (RCTs) have demonstrated that the CRC mortality can still be decreased in individuals who undergo routine FOBT. A positive FOBT needs to be further evaluated by direct visualization of the colon mucosa either via sigmoidoscopy, optical colonoscopy, or computed tomographic colonography (virtual colonoscopy).

Flexible sigmoidoscopy can allow for visualization of the distal colon up to the splenic flexure. Almost 50% of all colorectal tumors are within the reach of the sigmoidoscope. The test should be done at 5-year intervals, and a positive finding should be followed up by colonoscopy. Recent RCT data suggest even sigmoidoscopy can reduce morbidity and mortality from CRC.

Alternatively, optical colonoscopy allows for the direct visualization of the entire colonic mucosa and has a high sensitivity in detecting tumors. Because colonoscopy allows for the biopsy and excision of adenomatous lesions, it can reduce the incidence of cancer in screened individuals and is the preferred method of screening by most physicians. Computed tomographic colonography is a noninvasive alternative to colonoscopy that uses reconstructed computed tomography (CT) images to visualize the colon. Similar to optical colonoscopy, it requires bowel preparation and adequate distention of the colon for proper visualization. While there are no prospective studies demonstrating that virtual colonoscopy reduces CRC mortality, a recent trial comparing optical colonoscopy to virtual colonoscopy showed similar detection rates for advanced neoplasms. Finally, double-contrast barium enemas have been utilized to detect CRC. Unfortunately, the study is associated with a high false-negative rate due to misinterpretation, poor preparation, and difficulties in detecting smaller lesions. As a result, the use of this modality as a screening tool has been limited.

Adults who are at average risk for CRC have several options for screening. The American Cancer Society recommends CRC screening begin at age 50 and consist of annual FOBT with flexible sigmoidoscopy at 5-year intervals or optical colonoscopy at 10-year intervals. Individuals who are at higher risk of developing CRCs need to undergo a more rigorous evaluation. Individuals in whom there is a family history of CRC or adenomas in a first-degree relative before age 60 or in more than 2 first-degree family members of any age should undergo colonoscopy every 5 years starting at age 40 or 10 years prior to the youngest

| TABLE 24-1 | STAGING, TREATMENT SUMMARY, AND SURVIVAL RATES FOR COLORECTAL CARCINOMAS | | | | |
|---|---|---|---|---|---|
| TNM Stage | Primary Tumor* | Lymph Node Metastasis** | Distant Metastasis‡ | Treatment Modality | 5-year Survival |
| I | T1 or T2 | N0 | M0 | Surgery | 74% |
| II | T3 or T4 | N0 | M0 | Surgery +/- chemotherapy or chemo-radiotherapy (rectal tumors) | 37% to 67% |
| III | T1 or T2 T3 or T4 Any T | N1 N1 N2 | M0 M0 M0 | Surgery + chemotherapy or chemo-radiotherapy (rectal tumors) | 28% to 73% |
| IV | Any T | Any N | M1 | Chemotherapy | 6% |

*T1 indicates tumor invades submucosa; T2, tumor invades muscularis propria; T3, tumor invades through muscularis propria into subserosa or into nonperitoneal pericolic or perirectal tissues; T4, tumor perforates the visceral peritoneum or directly invades other organs or structures
**N0 indicates no regional lymph nodes; N1, metastases in 1 to 3 pericolic or perirectal lymph nodes; N2, metastases in 4 or more pericolic or perirectal lymph nodes
‡M0 indicates no distant metastasis; M1, distant metastasis
TNM indicates tumor, lymph node, metastases

relative diagnosed. In individuals who have CRC or adenomas in a first-degree family member at age 60 years or older, surveillance should begin with colonoscopy at age 40. Other high-risk individuals, such as those with genetic or clinical diagnosis of HNPCC (Lynch syndrome) should undergo colonoscopy every 1 to 1 years starting at age 20 to 25 years or 10 years before the earliest case in the immediate family.

## Treatment

Patients with localized CRC are primarily managed using a surgical approach. The need for pre- (neoadjuvant) or postoperative (adjuvant) chemotherapy with or without radiation is dependent on the location of the tumor (colon versus rectum) and the stage of the disease (Table 24-1). For colon tumors, the region of the bowel that contains the tumor, along with the associated mesentery and adjacent lymph nodes, are removed. Adequate lymph node dissection is vital for accurate staging and improved patient survival. It is recommended that a minimum of 12 lymph nodes be removed and available for evaluation by the pathologist. For rectal cancers, the procedure of choice is a total mesorectal excision (TME), in which the node bearing mesorectum surrounding the rectum is removed. Total mesorectal excision has been associated with significant reduction in local recurrence rates for patients with rectal cancers. Select patients with very small rectal tumors (<3 to 4 cm), with well- to moderately well-differentiated histology, and absence of lymphovascular invasion may be candidates for treatment by local excision alone.

Numerous clinical trials in the past decade have demonstrated the benefit of adjuvant chemotherapy in patients with lymph node-positive disease. 5-fluorouracil (5-FU) has been the backbone of adjuvant chemotherapy. Recently, the use of 5-FU, leucovorin, and oxaliplatin (FOLFOX regimen) was associated with improved disease-free survival and overall survival in patients with Stage III disease (MOSAIC Trial). As a result, FOLFOX is the recommended adjuvant treatment for patients with lymph node-positive colon cancer. For patients with Stage II resected disease, the benefit of chemotherapy is not as clear. The MOSAIC trial did include patients considered to be high-risk Stage II colon cancers, defined as having either a T4 lesion, perforation of bowel at presentation, peritumoral lymphovascular invasion, poorly differentiated on histology, or evidence for microsatellite instability (MSI). For such patients, an improvement in disease-free survival, but no overall survival benefit, was seen using adjuvant FOLFOX regimen.

In patients with rectal cancer, local recurrence in absence of metastatic disease is more common. Several studies have demonstrated the benefit of concurrent radiation therapy and chemotherapy in reducing the local recurrence rate as well as improving overall survival. For rectal cancers that approach the anal sphincter, neoadjuvant chemoradiation therapy allows for significant reduction of tumor size and allows for sphincter-preserving surgery. Furthermore, neoadjuvant therapy can reduce the long-term morbidity associated with radiation. Preoperative chemoradiation has been associated with lower local failure rate, high sphincter preservation, and lower incidence of anastomotic stricture. As a result, neoadjuvant therapy is now preferred in most cases, especially in patients with larger T3 or T4 tumors.

The primary treatment for advanced or metastatic CRC is systemic chemotherapy. Regimens using FOLFOX or 5-FU, leucovorin, and irinotecan (FOLFIRI) are frequently used as first or second lines of therapy in metastatic settings. The use of molecular targeted agents, such as the monoclonal antibodies bevacizumab (Avastin, Genentech, San Francisco, Calif) and cetuximab (Erbitux, ImClone LLC, New

York, NY), have improved the outcome for advanced CRC. Several clinical trials have demonstrated that addition of bevacizumab to systemic chemotherapy is associated with improvement in overall survival and response rate. In addition, cetuximab has been shown to also improve progression-free survival and response rates in select patients when used in conjunction with chemotherapy in first or subsequent lines of therapy.

## Surveillance

Upon completion of therapy for CRC, patients should undergo surveillance to monitor for post-therapy complications or development of recurrent disease. The National Cancer Comprehensive Network (NCCN) recommends patients be monitored with history and physical examination every 3 months for 2 years and then every 6 months for a total of 5 years. In addition, patients should undergo monitoring of carcinoembryonic antigen (CEA) levels at each visit. A colonoscopy should be performed 1 year from the date of surgery and should be repeated the following year if the results are abnormal, or at least every 2 to 3 years if results are positive for polyps. Patients should also undergo CT of the abdomen and pelvis along with chest x-ray every 6 months for the first 2 years and subsequently every 6 to 12 months for a total of 5 years.

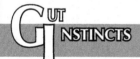

COLORECTAL CANCER

1. Optical colonoscopy is the preferred screening tool for most physicians.
2. Adequate lymph node dissection (12 lymph nodes) is critical for accurate staging and survival of locally advanced CRC.
3. 5-FU, leucovorin, and oxaliplatin (FOLFOX) is the recommended adjuvant chemotherapy regimen for lymph node-positive colon cancer.
4. Neoadjuvant chemoradiation is the treatment of choice for patients with T3 or T4 rectal tumors.
5. All resected patients with CRC should undergo screening colonoscopy 1 year postsurgery.

# Key References

1. Engstrom PF, Arnoletti JP, Benson AB, et al. Colon cancer–clinical practice guidelines in oncology. *J Natl Compr Canc Netw.* 2009;7(8):778-831.

2. Engstrom PF, Arnoletti JP, Benson AB, et al. Rectal cancer–clinical practice guidelines in oncology. *J Natl Compr Canc Netw.* 2009;7(8):838-881.

3. Levin B, Lieberman DA, McFarland B, et al. Screening and surveillance for the early detection of colorectal cancer and adenomatous polyps, 2008: a joint guideline from the American Cancer Society, the US Multi-Society Task Force on Colorectal Cancer, and the American College of Radiology. *CA Cancer J Clin.* 2008;58(3):130-160.

# CHAPTER 25

# COLON POLYPS

Eric Esrailian, MD, MPH

Although most colorectal polyps do not have any clinical significance, if a patient has polyps removed during an endoscopic procedure, a trajectory is often set for more frequent surveillance. The detection of polyps has implications for resource utilization, patient anxiety about the potential for colorectal cancer (CRC), and a potential impact on the screening of family members. Although many hyperplastic polyps have a characteristic appearance endoscopically, most endoscopists do not take chances and they take a "leave no polyp behind" approach. Ultimately, most colon cancers arise from adenomatous polyps. On the other hand, nonadenomatous polyps do not carry the same risk and do not warrant the same frequency of surveillance. Therefore, it is important to understand the significance of the different polyps removed during colonoscopy for surveillance intervals and risk assessments for CRC.

## Adenomatous Polyps

Essentially, these are the polyps that clinicians really care about, and most of them are sporadic. Adenocarcinoma of the colon is thought to generally progress via the adenoma-carcinoma sequence. Although colonoscopy is a critical method for CRC screening, it also serves a preventive role by allowing for the removal of adenomatous polyps. This removal has been shown to decrease the potential for colon cancer, and it is one of the few preventive mechanisms providers have. With suboptimal bowel preparations, diminutive lesions or flat lesions can be missed.

Esrailian E. *Gut Instincts: A Clinician's Handbook of Digestive and Liver Diseases* (pp 173-178).

## TUBULAR ADENOMAS

The great majority of adenomatous polyps are primarily tubular adenomas. By definition, all tubular adenomas have at least low-grade dysplasia, and there is a wide variation with respect to their prevalence. However, the prevalence increases with age. At an index colonoscopy, a tubular adenoma greater than 1 cm or the presence of 3 or more tubular adenomas is considered to carry a higher risk and to be more predictive of subsequent adenomas.

## TUBULOVILLOUS AND VILLOUS ADENOMAS

Villous architecture, regardless of the percentage, is now considered to be more advanced neoplasia. Although usually asymptomatic, villous adenomas can be symptomatic when large and can be associated with secretory diarrhea.

## SERRATED ADENOMAS

Although they have some overlapping features in terms of architecture, serrated polyps are distinct from hyperplastic polyps. CRC that develops from the serrated pathway is not thought to follow the same classic adenoma-carcinoma sequence. Traditional serrated adenomas, mixed serrated polyps, and sessile serrated adenomas are the subtypes, and the sessile serrated adenomas are the most common. The natural history of serrated adenomas is currently not well established, but even if dysplasia is not present, they should be managed in a similar fashion as conventional adenomas.

# Nonadenomatous Polyps

These polyps are typically less important clinically, with few exceptions. The distinction is important from a natural history perspective and from a resource utilization perspective in relation to surveillance colonoscopy.

## HYPERPLASTIC POLYPS

The majority of polyps in the colon are hyperplastic. In general, these polyps have no clinical significance and often are found in the sigmoid colon or rectum. Although many endoscopists feel comfortable distinguishing these polyps from adenomatous polyps endoscopically, histology is required to truly make this distinction. No surveillance is generally required for hyperplastic polyps, even if numerous polyps are present. However, hyperplastic polyposis syndrome is a rare syndrome in which there are numerous hyperplastic polyps, some of which are greater than 1 cm and spread throughout the colon. This syndrome is associated with a higher incidence of CRC, and an expedited surveillance interval is warranted.

## INFLAMMATORY POLYPS

These are polyps that result from chronic inflammation and can often be found in inflammatory bowel disease. Inflammatory polyps typically do not carry any malignant potential, but they may be difficult to distinguish from possible adenomatous polyps. They are also commonly seen at the site of surgical anastamoses. If a patient has numerous inflammatory polyps, accurate dysplasia surveillance via colonoscopy might not be possible.

## JUVENILE POLYPS

Juvenile polyps are hamartomas, lesions that arise from cells normally expected at those sites, and they are the most common polyps found in children. They are often pedunculated and asymptomatic. However, they can present with bleeding and can even prolapse out of the rectum. They are typically nondysplastic, but if part of the juvenile polyposis syndrome (more than 5 juvenile polyps present), they might be part of a familial condition.

# Polyposis Syndromes

Such syndromes are rare but are still encountered in clinical practice. They are associated with extracolonic malignancies as well, and clinicians should be aware of this potential. Among these rare syndromes, 2 that may be encountered in clinical practice are familial adenomatous polyposis (FAP) and Peutz-Jeghers syndrome (PJS).

## FAMILIAL ADENOMATOUS POLYPOSIS

This autosomal-dominant condition results from a mutation in the APC gene (chromosome 5) and is also called adenomatous polyposis coli. There is a 100% incidence of early colon cancer, and adenomatous polyps typically carpet the colon. An attenuated form of FAP exists with far fewer adenomas and a later progression to colon cancer. Even after colectomy, *surveillance upper endoscopy with side-viewing endoscopy* is required because peri-ampullary cancer is the second most common cancer detected in patients with FAP.

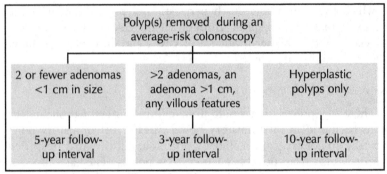

**Figure 25-1.** Polyp surveillance algorithm.

### PEUTZ-JEGHERS SYNDROME

This syndrome is rarer and is also an autosomal-dominant condition. However, it is associated with hamartomatous polyps. The classic muco-cutaneous pigmentation and melanin spots can usually be found in the perioral region. Peutz-Jeghers syndrome is associated with potential malignancies of the entire gastrointestinal tract, pancreas, cervix, ovary, and breast. Patients can present with small bowel polyps that result in intussusception or bleeding, and a small bowel evaluation should be considered endoscopically or with imaging in obscure or occult bleeding cases.

# Surveillance Practices: Shape, Size, and Location Matter

Once polyps have been detected, it is important to tailor a surveillance algorithm for each patient. Factors to consider include a patient's risk factors for colon cancer, polyp histology, and even the prep quality during the index colonoscopy. Synchronous lesions are those discovered during the same colonoscopy, whereas metachronous lesions are detected on subsequent procedures. Figure 25-1 outlines a surveillance algorithm for polyp surveillance in a patient with average risk. Expedited surveillance is not necessary for hyperplastic polyps in the absence of different clinical indications such as new bleeding and changes in bowel habits.

If polyps are sessile or removed piecemeal, endoscopic follow up might be necessary to ensure complete removal. Polyps are like real estate, and location is important. For distal lesions, short-term follow up can be performed with flexible sigmoidoscopy with minimal preparation. On the other hand, cecum or ascending colon lesions will require repeat colonoscopy. In either case, the patient's clinical status should always be assessed for safety and appropriateness. However, if incomplete removal of a right-sided polyp is suspected, an expedited colonoscopy should be recommended despite the possible inconvenience of a repeat bowel prep.

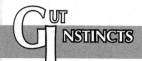

### COLON POLYPS

1. Hyperplastic polyps are generally insignificant. There is rarely any need for follow up with these more frequently in surveillance.

2. Large adenomas (>1 cm), multiple adenomas (>2 cm), any villous features, and high-grade dysplasia in a polyp are all considered higher risk situations and more predictive for future adenomatous polyps.

3. Serrated adenomas are distinct from hyperplastic polyps and should be managed as higher risk polyps with closer surveillance.

4. Patients with FAP should be screened for possible periampullary cancer using side-viewing endoscopy.

5. Flat polyps are not really always flat. They can be detected with a slow, careful withdrawal technique during a colonoscopy with an adequate bowel preparation.

## Key References

1. Brooks DD, Winawer SJ, Rex DK, et al. Colonoscopy surveillance after polypectomy and colorectal cancer resection. *Am Fam Physician*. 2008;77(7): 995-1002.

2. Bauer VP, Papaconstantinou HT. Management of serrated adenomas and hyperplastic polyps. *Clin Colon Rectal Surg*. 2008;21(4):273-279.

# CHAPTER 26

# CLOSTRIDIUM DIFFICILE

Theodoros Kelesidis, MD and
Charalabos Pothoulakis, MD

*Clostridium difficile* infection (CDI) represents the most common diarrheal infection in hospitals, affecting millions of patients annually in the United States and abroad. *C. difficile* has been identified as the pathogen causing pseudomembranous colitis and is emerging as one of the most significant hospital-acquired infections.

## Definition of *Clostridium difficile*

The diagnosis of CDI is based on a combination of clinical and laboratory findings. These include the passage of 3 or more unformed stools per day and a stool test result positive for the presence of *C. difficile* or its toxins. Less frequently, endoscopic or histopathologic findings demonstrating pseudomembranous colitis or a nonspecific colitis are associated with CDI. The disease severity of CDI is increasing, and a new virulent strain (eg, NAP 1/027) is emerging that is associated with increased morbidity and mortality.

## Microbiology and Pathogenicity

*C. difficile* is a gram-positive, spore-forming, anaerobic rod-shaped bacterium that is difficult to isolate in culture. The organism exists in a vegetative form, which is the most common and is highly sensitive to oxygen; or in spores, which are heat stable, resistant to the acidic environment of the stomach, and survive for long periods of time on

Esrailian E. *Gut Instincts: A Clinician's Handbook of Digestive and Liver Diseases* (pp 179-186).
© 2012 Taylor & Francis Group

hospital surfaces. *C. difficile* releases 2 potent exotoxins, toxin A and toxin B, that mediate the disease. The normal colonic microflora confers resistance against *C. difficile*. However, changes in the colonic microflora, most frequently by antibiotics, enable colonization with *C. difficile* leading to CDI.

## Epidemiology

*C. difficile* infection is primarily a nosocomial disease. The epidemiology of this disease is changing, and CDI is not considered a benign infection. The rates of CDI have almost doubled in the past 10 years, and *C. difficile* is the leading cause of antibiotic-associated diarrhea, accounting for approximately 15% to 25% of all episodes. This infection is associated with death in 0.6% to 1.5% of cases, and the 1-year CDI mortality rate has been described as high as 17%. In addition, CDI now involves patients previously thought to be at low risk and lacking the typical risk factors for infection. The reasons for this changing epidemiology include changes in antimicrobial use or infection control practices in hospitals, but most importantly, the emergence of the new, hypervirulent *C. difficile* strain that has become an epidemic in hospitals across the United States, Canada, and parts of Europe.

## Risk Factors

Antibiotic use is the main risk factor associated with CDI. Clindamycin, cephalosporins, penicillins, and fluoroquinolones are the most common antibiotics associated with CDI. However, virtually all antibacterial agents can cause CDI. Age (>65 years), chronic illnesses, increased length of hospital stays, and other conditions that may alter the bowel flora (eg, surgery, chemotherapy, or use of proton pump inhibitors [PPIs]) are also considered risk factors for CDI. Some measures to reduce hospital-acquired infections may actually increase the risk for *C. difficile*. While the use of alcohol-based hand sanitizers has been credited with reducing bacterial spread, it may not kill the spores, contributing to the spread of *C. difficile*.

## Clinical Presentation

*C. difficile* infection can occur as sporadic cases or nosocomial outbreaks. The primary symptoms are watery diarrhea, fever, abdominal pain, and/or tenderness. Patients may present with profound leukocytosis. The symptoms associated with CDI range from asymptomatic carriage to fulminant, life-threatening colitis (Table 26-1). Symptoms can appear during or immediately after antimicrobial therapy is initiated, or even several weeks (up to 90 days) after antibiotic intake.

| TABLE 26-1 | CLINICAL MANIFESTATIONS OF C. *DIFFICILE* INFECTION |
|---|---|
| **Clinical Type of C. *difficile* Infection** | **Comments** |
| Asymptomatic carriage | Approximately 3% to 5% of adults and 50% of neonates are asymptomatic carriers |
| | Approximately 25% to 30% of hospitalized adults are also C. *difficile* carriers |
| Mild-to-moderate diarrhea | One of the most common presentations of CDI |
| | Watery diarrhea |
| | Abdominal cramping may occur |
| | Patients do not appear toxic and systemic illness is not present |
| | Sigmoidoscopy usually does not reveal significant abnormalities |
| C. *difficile* colitis without pseudomembranes | Presence of fever, malaise, high-volume diarrhea, and moderate-to-severe abdominal pain |
| | Stools may have some trace blood |
| | Leukocytosis is common and may serve as a diagnostic clue |
| | On sigmoidoscopy, colitis is patchy and moderate; no pseudomembranes are present |
| Pseudomembranous colitis | Severe abdominal pain and tenderness, fever |
| | Severe diarrhea that may be bloody |
| | Marked elevations of the white blood cells in the range of 30 to 50 x 109/L may serve as a diagnostic clue |
| | Abdominal imaging reveals severe colonic edema/pancolitis |
| | Sigmoidoscopy shows the presence of pseudomembranes, which represent yellow inflammatory plaques |
| | Only about 10% involve the right side alone, are associated with ileus, but not diarrhea, and require colonoscopy |

(continued)

| TABLE 26-1 | CLINICAL MANIFESTATIONS OF C. *DIFFICILE* INFECTION (CONTINUED) |
|---|---|
| Clinical Type of C. *difficile* Infection | Comments |
| Acute abdomen with sepsis syndrome (toxic megacolon) | Fever, hypotension, and an acute abdomen; distention and rebound tenderness may be clinical findings |
| | Ileus, but not likely diarrhea |
| | Abdominal imaging reveals colonic dilatation/ megacolon |
| | Sigmoidoscopy or colonoscopy is relatively contraindicated |
| | Surgical consult should be obtained immediately |
| Recurrent CDI | 12% to 24% of patients develop a second episode of CDI within 2 months of the initial diagnosis |
| | If a patient has 2 or more episodes of CDI, the risk for recurrences increases to 50% to 65% |
| | Most patients with first-time relapse are successfully treated, and no further illness ensues |
| | A few cases have repeat relapses, which may be due to metronidazole resistance, reinfection, and/or persistence of spores in the gastrointestinal tract |

# Laboratory Detection

The cornerstone of laboratory diagnosis is the detection of toxins from fecal samples. Toxin enzyme immunoassays (EIA) are easier to perform and can be rapidly obtained but have lower sensitivity compared to the cell cytotoxicity assay or culture of toxigenic *C. difficile*. The cytotoxicity assay is considered the gold standard, but it requires specialized facilities. The latex agglutination test detects a clostridial protein, is rapid, and is very sensitive, but it detects both toxigenic and nontoxigenic *C. difficile* strains. A 2-step approach was recently recommended that includes an initial test with EIA or latex agglutination test, followed by confirmatory cytotoxicity assay or *C. difficile* culture. Real-time polymerase chain reaction (PCR) and fecal leukocyte testing may also help the diagnosis of CDI. It should be emphasized, however, that clinical CDI suspicion should always override negative laboratory results.

# Prevention

Prevention has 2 aspects: prevention of acquisition of *C. difficile,* and prevention of infection in colonized people. The most effective approach to decrease the spread of *C. difficile* is the combination of judicious use of antibiotics, vigilant hand hygiene, the use of isolation/ infection control practices, and use of various forms of environmental decontamination. Other ways of preventing CDI include limiting use of PPIs if not indicated. Although probiotics may have a place in preventing CDI, recent guidelines do not recommend their use to prevent primary CDI.

# Treatment of First Episode

For mere antibiotic-associated diarrhea, withdrawal of the suspected antibacterial agent may be sufficient to improve diarrheal symptoms. Stool for *C. difficile* toxin A and B should be ordered if CDI is suspected, and the clinical status should be monitored. For mild to moderate CDI, use of metronidazole (500 mg, 3 times daily; or 250 mg, 4 times daily, for 10 to 14 days) is recommended. In patients with severe CDI (see Table 26-1), treatment with oral vancomycin (125 mg orally, 4 times daily, for 10 to 14 days) is the therapy of choice. Antimotility agents should be avoided initially. Patients must be monitored for treatment failure, defined as no response after 1 week, although most patients show signs of improvement within 48 to 72 hours. If diarrhea persists, patients initially treated with metronidazole may be changed to vancomycin. For the treatment of severe, complicated CDI, oral vancomycin (500 mg, 4 times daily) with or without intravenously administered metronidazole (500 mg intravenously every 8 hours) should be considered. If ileus is present, vancomycin should be given rectally (500 mg in 100 mL of normal saline every 6 hours) as a retention enema. In severe disease, early recognition is critical, and surgery may be lifesaving. Subtotal colectomy, and preservation of the rectum, is a frequent operation of choice.

# Treatment of Recurrent *Clostridium difficile* Infection

The risk of recurrence of CDI after a single episode is high, with 8% to 50% of patients having at least a second episode after treatment with metronidazole or vancomycin. Treatment of the first recurrence should be with the same agent used for primary treatment. In second and subsequent recurrences, vancomycin is recommended. A different approach is needed for patients with multiple CDI recurrences, and observational studies have examined the use of long-term, tapering, or pulsed courses of vancomycin. Options for the treatment of relapsing CDI include intravenous immunoglobulin (400 mg/kg), fecal bacteriotherapy, rifampicin, probiotics, toxin-binding resins such cholestyramine or tolevamer, and experimental monoclonal antibodies against toxins A and B. Exciting evidence indicates that use of antitoxin monoclonal antibodies is associated with reduced relapsing rates. However, larger randomized clinical trials are needed to support these approaches.

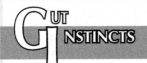

CLOSTRIDIUM DIFFICILE

1. Disease severity of CDI is increasing, and a new virulent strain associated with increased morbidity and mortality has emerged.

2. Virtually all antibacterial agents have been associated with CDI, and CDI is not only limited to broad-spectrum antibiotics.

3. The current cornerstone of laboratory diagnosis is the detection of toxin from fecal samples, with cell cytotoxicity assay representing the gold standard.

4. Prevention has 2 aspects (prevention of acquisition of C. difficile and prevention of infection in colonized people) and requires a multifaceted approach, including combination of judicious and appropriate use of antibiotics, vigilant hand hygiene, the use of isolation/infection control practices, and use of various forms of environmental decontamination.

5. The mainstay for treating CDI emphasizes supportive care, rehydration, withdrawal of the suspected causative agent, avoidance of antimotility agents, and use of antibiotics with activity against C. difficile (eg, metronidazole and vancomycin).

# Key References

1. Kelly CP, LaMont JT. *Clostridium difficile*—more difficult than ever. *N Engl J Med*. 2008;359(18):1932-1940.
2. Johnson S. Recurrent *Clostridium difficile* infection: a review of risk factors, treatment, and outcomes. *J Infect*. 2009;58(6):403-410.
3. Cohen SH, Gerding DN, Johnson S, et al. Clinical practice guidelines for *Clostridium difficile* infection in adults: 2010 update by the society for healthcare epidemiology of America (SHEA) and the infectious diseases society of America (IDSA). *Infect Control Hosp Epidemiol*. 2010;31(5):431-455.

# OTHER COMMON GASTROINTESTINAL INFECTIONS

David A. Pegues, MD

Acute gastroenteritis ranks second to acute respiratory illness among the most common diseases worldwide, and it is a frequent cause of childhood malnutrition and mortality. The annual rate of acute diarrheal illness ranges from 0.4 to 1.3 episodes per year among adults and 2 to 3 episodes per year in children in developed countries to up to 10 to 18 episodes per year among children in developing countries. In the United States, foodborne diseases account for approximately 76 million illnesses, 32,500 hospitalizations, and 5000 deaths annually.

## Etiology

Most cases of acute infectious gastroenteritis are probably viral, but bacterial causes are responsible for most cases of severe diarrhea (Figure 27-1). Protozoa are less commonly identified as the etiologic agents of acute gastrointestinal illness. The Centers for Disease Control and Prevention's FoodNet program estimated the 2009 annual incidence per 100,000 population by pathogen as follows: *Salmonella* (15.19), *Campylobacter* (13.02), *Shigella* (3.99), *Cryptosporidium* (2.86), Shiga toxin-producing *Escherichia coli* (STEC O157 0.99 and STEC non-O157 0.57), *Vibrio* (0.35), *Listeria* (0.34), *Yersinia* (0.32), and *Cyclospora* (0.07). The prevalence of infectious agents is vastly underestimated because many patients do not seek medical attention and testing is often not performed routinely.

Esrailian E. *Gut Instincts: A Clinician's Handbook of Digestive and Liver Diseases* (pp 187-192).

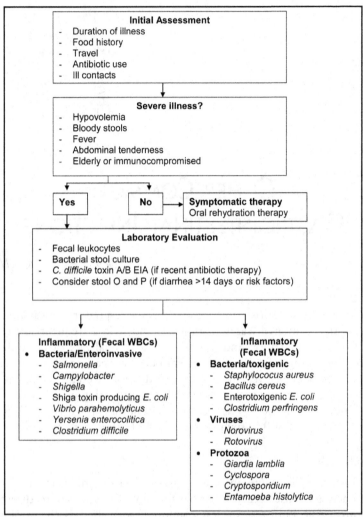

**Figure 27-1.** Evaluation of acute gastroenteritis.

# Diagnostic Approach

The initial evaluation of patients with acute diarrhea (≤14 days duration) should include looking for signs of intravascular volume depletion (eg, decreased skin turgor, orthostatic hypotension), fever, and peritoneal signs (see Figure 27-1). Travel history and food history should be obtained, including consumption of raw or undercooked meats, eggs, seafood, shellfish, and unpasteurized dairy products. It is also important to ask about recent antibiotic use and whether there is any history of immunosuppression, including pregnancy and human immunodeficiency virus (HIV), which increases the risk and severity of infection with *Listeria* and *Salmonella*, respectively.

Timing of symptom onset following ingestion of a suspected food item is important. Symptoms beginning within 6 hours of exposure suggest ingestion of a preformed toxin (*Bacillus cereus* or *Staphylococcus aureus*), and onset within 8 to 12 hours suggests *Clostridium perfringens*. Most other bacterial or viral causes have incubation periods of 1 to 3 days.

Several features can aid in distinguishing viral from bacterial causes of gastroenteritis. Viral gastroenteritis is more common in the winter months, is often accompanied by vomiting, and diarrhea is almost always nonbloody. Noroviruses affect all ages and are responsible for approximately 50% of all episodes of acute gastroenteritis. Other common causes of viral gastroenteritis (rotovirus, adenovirus, astrovirus) predominantly affect children younger than 5 years of age.

Most infectious causes of acute diarrhea are self-limited. Diagnostic evaluation, including examination of the stool for fecal leukocytes and bacterial stool culture, is indicated for patients with more severe illness, with at least one of the following signs or symptoms:

- Hypovolemia/orthostatic hypotension
- Bloody diarrhea (suggests Shiga toxin-producing *Escherichia coli* [STEC] and less commonly *Shigella*, *Campylobacter*, and *Salmonella*)
- Temperature 38.5°C or higher (101.3°F)
- Passage of 6 or more unformed stools in 24 hours
- Duration of illness longer than 48 hours
- Severe abdominal pain
- Recent use of antibiotics or hospitalized patients
- Diarrhea in elderly patients (70 years of age or older) or immunocompromised patients

## EXAMINATION OF STOOL FOR FECAL LEUKOCYTES

The sensitivity and specificity of fecal leukocytes for inflammatory/infectious diarrhea has been estimated at 70% and 50% to 80%, respectively, and supports the diagnosis of a bacterial cause of diarrhea in patients with severe illness. It is of limited value in patients who develop diarrhea following hospitalization, where a stool assay for *C. difficile* toxin should be performed.

## ROUTINE STOOL CULTURE

Stool cultures for bacterial pathogens are infrequently positive (<6%) except in patients with severe disease where yield may approach 85%. Routine stool culture will identify *Salmonella, Campylobacter,* and *Shigella,* the most common bacterial causes of gastroenteritis, as well as *Aeromonas* and *Yersenia* species. The laboratory must be notified if infection with *Listeria* or STEC is suspected.

## STOOL EXAMINATION FOR OVA AND PARASITES

Stool examination for ova and parasites should be reserved for patients with persistent diarrhea (>14 days), especially when there is a history of the following:

- Travel to mountainous regions, Russia, or Nepal (*Giardia*)
- Exposure to infants in daycare or a community waterborne outbreak (*Giardia* and *Cryptosporidium*)
- Men who have sex with men (*Giardia* and *Entamaeba histolytica*)
- Persons with HIV/acquired immune deficiency syndrome (*Cryptosporidium, Isospora, Cyclospora, Microsporidia*)
- Patients with bloody diarrhea with few/no fecal leukocytes (*E. histolytica*).

Three specimens should be collected at least 24 hours apart because excretion of parasites may be intermittent. Specific testing of stool must be requested for *Giardia* and *Cryptosporidium* (by direct immunofluorescence) and *Cyclospora* and *Isospora* (by modified acid fast staining).

## VIRAL DETECTION

*Rotovirus* can be directly detected in fresh stool specimens by enzyme immunoassay, latex agglutination, or polymerase chain reaction (PCR). Testing for norovirus by PCR of stool or vomitus is usually reserved for outbreak situations.

# Empiric Treatment

Rehydration, preferably with oral rehydration solution containing water, salt, and sugar, is the most critical therapy. Sports drinks for sweat replacement (eg, Gatorade, The Gatorade Company, Chicago, IL) are not equivalent to oral rehydration solution. Antibiotic therapy is not required in most cases of acute gastroenteritis because the illness is usually self-limited and therapy does not significantly alter the course of illness in unselected populations. Antibiotics should be avoided in patients with suspected or confirmed enterohaemorrhagic *E. coli* infection because they may increase the risk of hemolytic uremic syndrome.

Empiric antibiotic therapy should be considered in the following groups:

- Those with moderate to severe travelers' diarrhea with more than 4 unformed stools per day with fever, blood, or mucus in the stool.

- Those with more than 8 stools per day, volume depletion, symptoms for more than 1 week, immunocompromised hosts, or those in whom hospitalization is being considered.

If empiric antibiotic therapy is warranted, an oral fluoroquinolone should be administered for 3 to 5 days, such as ciprofloxacin 500 mg twice daily, norfloxacin 400 mg twice daily, or levofloxacin 500 mg once daily. Fluoroquinolone resistance is uncommon among enteric bacterial pathogens except for *Campylobacter*.

## Directed Treatment

If fluoroquinolone-resistant *Campylobacter* is suspected (eg, foreign travel or failure of empiric fluoroquinolone therapy) or confirmed by susceptibility testing, azithromycin 500 mg once daily for 3 days should be given. The treatment of *C. difficile* infection is discussed in Chapter 26. Agents active against selected protozoal causes of gastroenteritis include metronidazole (*E. histolytica, Giardia, Cryptosporidium*), trimethoprim/sulfamethoxazole (*Isospora, Cyclospora*), albendazole (*Microsporidium*), and nitazoxanide and paromomycin (*Cryptosporidium*).

## Symptomatic Therapy and Diet

Antimotility agents (eg, loperamide 4 mg initially then 2 mg after each unformed stool for ≤2 days; maximal daily dose, 16 mg) should be considered only for patients with diarrhea that lasts more than 2 days with no fever and nonbloody stools. Loperamide is more rapidly effective than bismuth subsalicylate. Probiotics, including *Saccharomyces, Lactobacillus,* and *Bifidobacterium*, are useful for the prevention and treatment of travelers' diarrhea. *Lactobacillus* modestly shortens the duration of illness and frequency of diarrhea in children with presumed viral gastroenteritis. Because secondary lactose intolerance may be common after acute gastroenteritis, temporary avoidance of lactose-containing foods may be considered.

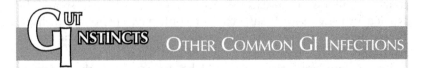

1. The initial evaluation of patients with acute diarrhea (≤14 days duration) should include a careful history and examination for fever, evidence of volume depletion, and peritoneal signs that suggest an invasive enteric bacterial infection.

2. Stool samples for evaluation for fecal leukocytes and bacterial culture should be obtained in patients with more severe illness or who are immunocompromised.

3. Stool examination for ova and parasites should not be obtained routinely, but should be considered in patients with persistent diarrhea (>14 days) and other risk factors.

4. Management of patients with gastroenteritis should first focus on hydration using oral rehydration solutions. Antimotility agents can be used in selected patients with diarrhea for more than 2 days with no fever and nonbloody stools.

5. Empiric antibiotic therapy with a fluoroquinolone for 3 to 5 days should be considered for patients with severe travelers' diarrhea or severe gastroenteritis, but not if suspected or confirmed enterohaemorrhagic E. coli infection exists because of the risk of hemolytic uremic syndrome.

## Key References

1. Al-Abri S, Beeching NJ, Nye FJ. Traveler's diarrhea. *Lancet Infect Dis.* 2005;5(6):349-360.

2. Glass RI, Parashar UD, Estes MK. Norovius gastroenteritis. *N Engl J Med.* 2009;361(18):1776-1785.

3. Musher DM, Musher BL. Contagious acute gastrointestinal infections. *N Engl J Med.* 2004;351(23):2417-2427.

4. Sazawal S, Hiremath G, Dhingra U, Malik P, Deb S, Black R. Efficacy of probiotics in prevention of acute diarrhea: a meta-analysis of masked, randomized, placebo controlled trials. *Lancet Infect Dis.* 2006;6(6):374-382.

# CHAPTER 28

# ILEUS AND BOWEL OBSTRUCTION

Lilah F. Morris, MD and
O. Joe Hines, MD

Ileus and bowel obstruction exist along a spectrum of gut motility disorders and present with nausea, abdominal distention, and obstipation. Sometimes, they are difficult to distinguish radiographically. However, the etiology and, therefore, treatment strategy for each are divergent. Ileus represents delayed motility and intestinal distention in the absence of mechanical obstruction, often occurring secondary to an underlying inflammatory process. Its resolution is dictated by the outcome of the inciting event. Bowel obstruction, caused by an intraluminal or extrinsic process that mechanically impedes intestinal transit, has a range of presentations from mild, self-limited abdominal discomfort to overt ischemia or perforation of the bowel.

## Ileus

Sometimes described as paralytic, ileus is a functional gut motility disorder. Ileus most commonly occurs in the postoperative setting secondary to bowel edema and inflammation from the surgical procedure, narcotic use, and electrolyte abnormalities due to lack of normal food intake. Ileus resolves and bowel motility typically returns within 2 to 4 days postoperatively, but can take as long as 1 week. Patients also develop ileus in the face of systemic (diabetic ketoacidosis), localized abdominal (pancreatitis), or pelvic (pelvic inflammatory disease) pathologic processes.

Esrailian E. *Gut Instincts: A Clinician's Handbook of Digestive and Liver Diseases* (pp 193-198).
© 2012 Taylor & Francis Group

| TABLE 28-1 | CAUSES OF ILEUS AND BOWEL OBSTRUCTION |
|---|---|
| **Causes of Ileus** | **Causes of Bowel Obstruction** |
| Metabolic<br>• Hypokalemia<br>• Hypomagnesemia<br>• Hyponatremia<br>• Uremia<br>• Diabetic ketoacidosis<br>• Hyperparathyroidism<br><br>Neurogenic<br>• Postoperative<br>• Drugs (opioid narcotics, psychotropic agents)<br>• Spinal cord injury | Intraluminal<br>• Foreign body<br>• Bezoar<br>• Inspissated feces<br>• Gallstone ileus<br>• Intussusception<br>• Congenital atresia, stricture, or stenosis<br>• Meckel's diverticulum<br>• Crohn's disease strictures<br>• Diverticulitis<br>• Radiation enteritis<br>• Neoplasm<br>• Polypoid lesion<br>• Traumatic (mural hematoma) |
| Infection<br>• Systemic sepsis<br>• Pancreatitis<br>• Intra-abdominal abscess<br>• Peritonitis<br><br>Inflammation<br>• Retroperitoneal hemorrhage or inflammation<br>• Intra-abdominal inflammation (pancreatitis, hemorrhage) | Extrinsic<br>• Adhesions (typically postoperative)<br>• Hernia<br>• Congenital Ladd's bands<br>• Postinflammatory<br>• Volvulus<br>• Neoplasm causing external compression<br>• Annular pancreas<br>• Carcinomatosis<br>• Endometriosis |

## CLINICAL PRESENTATION

Ileus and bowel obstruction may have a strikingly similar presentation and have multiple causes (Table 28-1). Colicky abdominal pain, abdominal distention, nausea, vomiting, and failure to pass flatus or feces are typical subjective complaints, although many of these may be absent. A careful history might elicit recent abdominal surgery or an underlying intra-abdominal process like acute cholecystitis. In the immediate postoperative setting, ileus is the most likely diagnosis in patients with the described symptoms. In other contexts, it is a diagnosis of exclusion.

Physical examination findings include abdominal distention with the absence of bowel sounds on auscultation. Abdominal tenderness may be absent, but if detected, it is typically diffuse and mild. These patients do not exhibit signs of peritonitis like guarding or rebound.

## LABORATORY AND RADIOGRAPHIC ANALYSIS

Upright abdominal radiographs are the first imaging studies that should be obtained. An abdominal series includes a supine abdominal radiograph as well as upright abdominal and chest x-rays. Most patients with an intra-abdominal process, including infection, inflammation, or bleeding, will have dilated loops of bowel (>3 cm) on abdominal x-ray. Small bowel dilation is limited in ileus; dilation of more than 4 cm may indicate a mechanical obstruction. Additionally, this distended gas pattern is more likely to indicate an ileus if the air is distributed throughout the small bowel and colon rather than the distension in a proximal segment of bowel without distal bowel air.

Clues to the underlying inflammatory response causing bowel dilation may not be present on plain radiographs, leading the physician to pursue a computed tomography (CT) scan. This imaging modality can help identify an etiology of the ileus or may help distinguish it from a mechanical obstruction. A CT scan is also helpful in evaluation of prolonged postoperative ileus to eliminate abscess or infection as a source of delayed gut motility.

## MANAGEMENT

The management of ileus is supportive, with intravenous fluids and nasogastric tube decompression, while treatment is provided for the underlying disease process. Electrolyte abnormalities should be aggressively corrected and medications causing bowel dysmotility discontinued. While the use of various prokinetic agents has been advocated in some studies, none of these have demonstrated enough effectiveness to be used routinely.

Acute colonic pseudo-obstruction, or Ogilvie's syndrome, deserves mention. This clinical disorder presents with signs and symptoms of large bowel obstruction in the absence of a mechanical cause. The classic presentation is an elderly patient with multiple comorbid conditions, presenting with abdominal pain, nausea, vomiting, abdominal distention, and a dilated colon on abdominal radiographs. Both the acetylcholinesterase inhibitor neostigmine (while on cardiac monitor) and enemas have been successful medical treatments if the patient is clinically stable and decompression is not pursued. However, risk of perforation accompanies this disorder, and colon dilation more than 10 cm should lead to emergent colonoscopic decompression or surgical intervention.

# Bowel Obstruction

The most common causes of bowel obstruction in the United States are adhesions, hernias, and malignancy. Obstructions are classified according to location along the gastrointestinal tract and whether the obstruction is partial (bowel lumen is narrowed) or complete (lumen is totally obstructed). The former are more likely than the latter to resolve with conservative management. Open-loop obstructions refer to bowel tethered in one location, and proximal and distal decompression is possible. Closed-loop obstructions refer to torsion of the bowel around an adhesive band, volvulus, or internal hernia and lead to a segment of bowel with compromised vascular perfusion.

## CLINICAL PRESENTATION

The presentation of bowel obstruction varies widely. In early or self-limited obstruction, patients complain of abdominal discomfort, distention, and failure of passage of flatus and feces. Diarrhea may occur secondary to increased contractile activity as the liquid content of the stool is propelled past the point of obstruction. Nausea and vomiting indicate a more proximal obstruction. The time course of symptoms varies widely; patients with complete obstruction will present with near-immediate symptoms, whereas patients with chronic large bowel obstruction from diverticulitis may present with several weeks of abdominal distention. A history of prior abdominal or pelvic infections, surgery, or malignancy might be apparent.

Physical examination will reveal normal vital signs with diffuse abdominal tenderness in patients with early obstruction, progressing to intense, unremitting abdominal pain and overt signs of sepsis (eg, fever, tachycardia, hypotension) in patients with complete obstruction and ischemic bowel. A search for the presence of surgical scars and inguinal or femoral hernias should be undertaken. Rectal examination is mandatory to eliminate fecal impaction or very distal obstruction as an etiology and to identify bleeding, which may indicate intestinal ischemia.

## LABORATORY AND RADIOGRAPHIC ANALYSIS

Evaluation of a patient with suspected bowel obstruction should include a full laboratory panel including electrolytes and complete blood count. Leukocytosis, metabolic acidosis, and elevated lactate are signs of ischemia. Dehydration often accompanies the presentation of bowel obstruction, and blood urea nitrogen and creatinine levels should be compared to baseline.

Plain films can reveal the extent of obstruction and should always be undertaken first. Gas visualized in the rectum virtually excludes the diagnosis. Large, dilated loops of bowel and air fluid levels are visualized. CT scans can be both diagnostic and therapeutic. Initially, they can help identify a precise transition point in the bowel but are most useful to determine the presence of complete obstruction that requires urgent operative intervention. In addition, ingestion of hypertonic, water-soluble contrast (gastrograffin) has been shown in several studies to be therapeutic in the setting of partial bowel obstruction. These agents cause a shift of fluid into the intestinal lumen and increase the pressure gradient across the site of obstruction.

## MANAGEMENT

Bowel obstruction can be life threatening. The most critical treatment decisions involve recognition of patients who can tolerate observation versus those who require emergent surgical intervention. All patients require supportive care with intravenous fluid resuscitation and nasogastric tube decompression. The presence of peritonitis, fevers, tachycardia, or hypotension, as well as any radiographic evidence of a closed-loop obstruction, requires emergent operative exploration. Patients who are initially managed with observation should be assiduously monitored for signs of bowel compromise. If patients fail to progress with observation after a period of 3 to 5 days, re-evaluation with CT scan or operative intervention is warranted. Patients in whom operative management should be avoided are those with early postoperative bowel obstruction, obstruction in the setting of Crohn's disease, and carcinomatosis. Patients with single-band adhesions, limited abdominal distension, and partial bowel obstruction who are clinically stable may be candidates for laparoscopic enterolysis. However, generally, exploration is undertaken via laparotomy.

## Gut Instincts  ILEUS AND BOWEL OBSTRUCTION

1. Ileus is a functional gut motility disorder occurring in the absence of mechanical obstruction and arising in the postoperative state or from an underlying inflammatory process. Bowel obstruction represents delayed gut motility secondary to a mechanical blockage.

2. Management of ileus is medical, with intravenous fluid resuscitation and nasogastric tube decompression, while a search and treatment of the underlying etiology is undertaken.

3. Partial and open-loop bowel obstructions can be treated conservatively with frequent reassessment for signs of progression.

4. Plain abdominal x-rays should be obtained first in assessment for both ileus and bowel obstruction, with CT scans used secondarily if additional information related to the etiology and presence of closed-loop obstruction is required.

5. Bowel obstruction that presents with constant abdominal pain, marked tenderness, leukocytosis, and metabolic acidosis likely represents closed-loop obstruction or ischemic bowel and requires aggressive resuscitation and emergent surgical intervention.

## Key References

1. Diaz JJ Jr, Bokhari F, Mowery NT, et al. Guidelines for management of small bowel obstruction. *J Trauma*. 2008;64(6):1651-1664.

2. Story SK, Chamberlin RS. A comprehensive review of evidence-based strategies to prevent and treat post-operative ileus. *Dig Surg*. 2009;26(4):265-275.

# CHAPTER 29

# HEMORRHOIDS

Jonathan Sack, MD

## Presentation and Diagnosis

Hemorrhoids are a normal anatomic structure that commonly become pathologically enlarged and produce a variety of symptoms. Due to a variety of stresses, including upright posture and an omnivorous diet, the 3 hemorrhoidal sinusoidal tufts (left lateral, right anterior, and right posterior) become dilated due to arteriovenous malformations producing engorgement with resultant redundancy of the overlying mucosa. These sagging internal hemorrhoids can prolapse into or through the anal canal and become symptomatic. Prolapsing internal hemorrhoids can cause anal leakage by preventing closure of the anal canal. The resultant fecal soilage can cause perianal skin irritation sometimes perceived as itching or pruritis ani. Painless, episodic bright red rectal bleeding is a common symptom of diseased internal hemorrhoids and is induced by minor trauma during defecation, producing a mucosal erosion overlying an engorged internal hemorrhoidal sinusoidal complex. The bleeding occurs with defecation, often is present in the toilet bowl or on the paper, and is bright red due to the arterial nature of the mucosal erosion. The bleeding is usually self-limited and rarely produces anemia, tachycardia, or hypotension. It is essential not to dismiss rectal bleeding as simply from hemorrhoids because rectal bleeding is the most common presenting symptom of colon and rectal cancer. Although some information can be inferred from the character of the

Esrailian E. *Gut Instincts: A Clinician's Handbook of Digestive and Liver Diseases* (pp 199-204). © 2012 Taylor & Francis Group bleeding, the clinician must maintain a high index of suspicion for possible malignancy. Patients often become alarmed by the seemingly voluminous amount of blood because a small amount of blood can turn the entire toilet bowl red. Anticoagulation with aspirin, clopidrogrel (Plavix), or warfarin (Coumadin) may exacerbate the bleeding. Pain is another common symptom of hemorrhoids and is commonly perceived as a pressure sensation because the stretch receptors found above the dentate line lack a somatic component.

## Treatment of Internal Hemorrhoids

Symptomatic internal hemorrhoids can be treated conservatively with a high-fiber diet, bulk supplements such as psyllium (Metamucil, Procter & Gamble, Cincinnati, OH), methylcellulose (Citrucel, Bayer HealthCare LLC, Morristown, NJ), or calcium polycarbophil (FiberCon, Pfizer, New York, NY), stool softeners such as docusate sodium (Colace, Purdue Pharma LP, Stamford, CT), and topical preparations containing hydrocortisone and a topical analgesic (Analpram, Ferndale Pharma Group, Inc, Ferndale, MI) or similarly composed suppositories (Anusol-HC, Salix Pharmaceuticals, Morrisville, NC). Office-based, nonoperative treatment of internal hemorrhoids may be performed for bleeding, pain, protrusion, leakage, and itching. All treatments of internal hemorrhoids depend on submucosal fibrosis to extrinsically compress the hemorrhoidal sinusoids. Induction of scar may be achieved by rubberband ligation, injection sclerosis (with sodium morrhuate or phenol), infrared coagulation, and cauterization with monopolar (Ultroid, Ultroid Technologies, Inc, Tampa, FL) or bipolar cautery (Bicap, Conmed Corporation, Utica, NY). Excisional hemorrhoidectomy is reserved for severe cases or those not responding to nonoperative treatment. Although the results of hemorrhoid treatment are good, recurrence is common, and the treatment may need to be repeated. Stapled hemorrhoidopexy (Procedure for Prolapse and Hemorrhoids [PPH]) and Doppler-guided selective dearterialization are newer modalities of treatment with less postoperative pain but are only applicable in selected individuals with isolated internal hemorrhoids because the external component is not effectively treated with these procedures. All hemorrhoidectomy specimens are sent for routine pathology because anal malignancy may occasionally masquerade as internal hemorrhoids. Incarcerated prolapsed internal hemorrhoids are a special circumstance requiring emergency treatment. Strangulation can result in thrombosis and ischemic necrosis with ulceration and suppuration. Emergent treatment involves reduction under anesthesia and emergency hemorrhoidectomy.

It is important to distinguish the protrusion of prolapsing internal hemorrhoids, which produce radial folds, from the circular folds seen with complete rectal prolapse. Complete rectal prolapse (procidentia) is a rectal intussusception that requires 3 prerequisites: (1) a permissive anal sphincter; (2) failure of the pelvic floor; and (3) a redundant rectosigmoid mesentery and deep cul-de-sac. These conditions occur most often in postpartum women but may occur in nulliparous women or rarely in men if the pelvic floor is dysfunctional due to repeated mechanical stress such as a chronic cough, straining, chronic constipation, or neurogenic causes. Surgical treatment of complete rectal prolapse is indicated for symptoms such as pain, bleeding, and anal leakage. Emergent operation is sometimes necessary for incarcerated or strangulated prolapse. Surgery for complete rectal prolapse involves removal of the redundant colon with rectal fixation. This may be accomplished through a laparoscopic or open abdominal procedure (resection-rectopexy or Goldman-Frykberg procedure), a perineal procedure, such as perineal mucosal proctectomy (Delorme procedure), or perineal proctectomy (Altemeier procedure). Anal continence and defecatory function are not always restored after surgery because of the underlying pelvic floor dysfunction, but symptoms such as bleeding, pain, mucoid discharge, and protrusion may be relieved. Other manifestations of pelvic floor dysfunction may be present, such as cystocele, enterocele, rectocele, and uterine prolapse. A multidisciplinary approach to these conditions is often indicated, involving the disciplines of urology, gynecology, and colon and rectal surgery or a pelvic floor reconstructive surgeon with specialized training in all of these areas.

## Treatment of External Hemorrhoids

Thrombosed external hemorrhoids present as an acutely painful perianal mass that is tender to the touch. The pain may be severe enough to produce obstipation and urinary retention. The inflammatory response to the thrombosis and extravasated blood produces swelling over the ensuing several days that may be severe enough to cause ischemic necrosis of the overlying skin with ulceration and possible abscess formation. Emergent treatment of acutely thrombosed hemorrhoids may require local excision of the thrombosed vein. Incision and extrusion of the clot from an acutely thrombosed hemorrhoid should be avoided because recurrence is common if the vein is not excised. The pain of the excision is sometimes equivalent to the pain of the thrombosis, and intervention should be judiciously applied for selected patients in the first 48 hours, after which adhesion and perihemorrhoidal inflammation make excision treacherous. Local treatment consists of application of a topical astringent, such as witch hazel (Tuck's Medicated Pads, McNeil PPC, Skillman, NJ), as well as moist heat and nonsteroidal anti-inflammatory drugs (NSAIDs). NSAIDs are analgesic, anti-inflammatory, and anti-platelet, and this reduces the risk of recurrent thrombosis. With local treatment, the symptoms usually subside after 72 hours. Hemorrhoidectomy should not be performed in patients with Crohn's disease because healing is impaired and anorectal fistula or nonhealing wounds with discharge or incontinence are common complications. Care must be taken never to cut the anal sphincter in patients with inflammatory bowel disease because incontinence may occur. These patients may require proctocolectomy and ileostomy for complications of anorectal Crohn's or its treatment.

## Skin Tags

Skin tags are a common sequelae of external hemorrhoids and represent residual excess skin from stretching following an episode of acute thrombosis. There is always a subjacent submucosal hemorrhoidal vein beneath the skin tag, and these may undergo recurrent thrombosis. Small skin tags are usually asymptomatic. Larger skin tags can produce difficult anal hygiene with difficulty cleansing and may cause perianal skin irritation. In addition, the base of a large skin tag may tear from traction and produce an acutely painful fissure of the anoderm. Development of these symptoms is an indication for surgical removal of anal skin tags. Simple elliptical excision of the excess skin and subjacent hemorrhoid is effective, but it produces significant disability in the postoperative period due to pain from the perianal wound. Complications include infection, abscess formation, wound dehiscence with secondary healing, and recurrent skin tag formation with deformity of the perianal skin. Anal stenosis may occur if the excision is excessive.

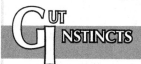

**HEMORRHOIDS**

1. Symptomatic hemorrhoids are a common affliction. While most hemorrhoids require treatment, few require surgery.
2. If urgent treatment of an acutely thrombosed external hemorrhoid is necessary, excision of the vein is preferred over extrusion of the clot.
3. Hemorrhoids cannot be permanently eradicated.
4. The best local treatment of a thrombosed external hemorrhoid consists of application of a topical astringent, moist heat, and NSAIDs.
5. Hemorrhoidectomy should not be performed in patients with Crohn's disease.

## Key Reference

1. Billingham RP, Isler JT, Kimmins MH, et al. The diagnosis and management of common anorectal problems. *Curr Probl Surg.* 2004;41(7):586-645.

# CHAPTER 30

# FISSURES, FISTULAE, AND CONDYLOMA

Jonathan Sack, MD

## Anal Fissure

### PRESENTATION AND DIAGNOSIS

Anal fissure is a radial tear in the anoderm that occurs due to local trauma, most commonly, passage of a large, hard stool. Painful defecation, often with bleeding, is characteristic. There can be both an initial sharp pain with hematochezia and a postdefecatory spastic pain, which can persist for several hours. Spasm of the internal anal sphincter produces relative cutaneous ischemia, which impairs healing. Most acute anal fissures heal spontaneously, but if an acute fissure fails to heal within 6 weeks, it is termed a *chronic anal fissure*. Approximately 90% of typical anal fissures are located within 90 degrees of the posterior midline. Anterior fissures are more common in postpartum women and may be ischemic in origin. Sometimes, the secondary opening of an anorectal fistula may be confused with an anal fissure, except for the presence of a tender crypt at the dentate line. Fissures may be diagnosed by eliciting a careful history and may be detected by external visual examination using eversion of the perianal skin to demonstrate the tear just inside the anal verge. Additional diagnostic features include a sentinel skin tag external to the fissure or a hypertrophic anal papillae internal to the fissure. No further examination is warranted once a fissure is detected because this is usually poorly tolerated. If a fissure

Esrailian E. *Gut Instincts: A Clinician's Handbook of Digestive and Liver Diseases* (pp 205-210).
© 2012 Taylor & Francis Group

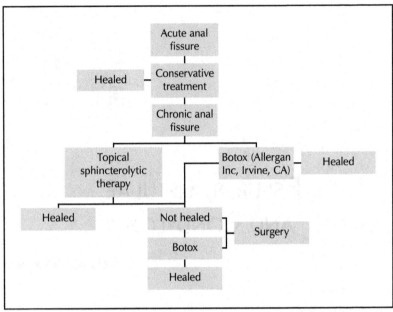

**Figure 30-1.** Treatment of acute anal fissure.

is chronic, digital examination after application of a topical local anesthetic may reveal internal anal sphincter spasm or even loss of normal anal canal dispensability, indicating chronic fibrosis of the internal anal sphincter with anal stenosis.

## TREATMENT

Treatment of anal fissure (Figure 30-1) is directed toward relaxation of the internal anal sphincter. This can be accomplished to some degree with local heat, such as hot water soaks, especially after defecation. Topical sphincterolytics are usually prescribed and include calcium channel blockers (diltiazem or verapamil) or a nitric oxide donor (nitroglycerin) compounded either as an ointment or a cream. These agents act locally by transdermal absorption. Some patients are intolerant of nitroglycerin due to headache. Ancillary measures include stool softeners such as docusate and topical anesthetics. Anal hygiene measures include avoiding alcohol or witch hazel and instead using baby wipes, moistened toilet paper, or a bidet after defecation. A lubricant/irritant laxative such as mineral oil (Kondremul, Heritage Brands Insight Pharmaceuticals Corp, Langhorne, PA) or an osmotic laxative, such as

Miralax (Schering-Plough HealthCare Products, Inc, Memphis, TN), may be helpful to prevent further constipation. Narcotics should be avoided to prevent constipation but may be necessary if pain is severe. Nonsteroidal anti-inflammatory drugs and acetaminophen may also help diminish pain. A high-fiber diet or fiber supplements may help maintain regularity, but they can also exacerbate pain by producing bulky stools. The rate of healing for chronic anal fissures with topical sphincterolytic therapy is approximately 60%, and crossover from one drug class to another can enhance the healing rate. Failure to heal or improve after 3 months of topical sphincterolytic therapy is an indication for injection of botulism toxin (Botox, Allergan Inc, Irvine, CA) into the intersphincteric groove to reversibly paralyze the internal anal sphincter for up to 3 months. Approximately 60% of chronic anal fissures refractory to topical sphincterolytic therapy will heal with Botox injection. Failure to heal after Botox injection is usually treated by a second Botox injection or surgery. Surgical treatment involves partial internal anal sphincterotomy with or without fissurectomy and anoplasty advancement flap closure of the fissure. Following partial internal anal sphincterotomy, there is a 90% rate of healing, but there is a 10% risk of gaseous incontinence.

# Cryptoglandular Diseases: Perirectal Abscess and Anorectal Fistula

## PRESENTATION AND DIAGNOSIS

The junction of the rectum with the anal canal is surrounded by 8 to 12 anal crypts, which are the openings for the anal glands. Anal glands are pheromone-secreting glands undergoing evolutionary regression, and obstruction of the crypt opening can produce accumulation of secretions with bacterial infection termed *anal cryptitis*. Anal cryptitis may present as chronic anal pain of unknown etiology and is diagnosed by a subtle depression palpable at the dentate line with associated point tenderness. Unroofing of the offending crypt often relieves the chronic pain. Anal cryptitis may progress to perirectal abscess due to burrowing of the infectious tract circumferentially, proximally, distally, and radially in three dimensions. This may produce perianal abscess, ischiorectal fossa abscess, or supralevator abscess if the tract is intersphincteric, trans-sphincteric, or suprasphincteric, respectively. Presenting signs and symptoms of perirectal abscess include pain, swelling, erythema, induration, and fluctuance with purulent drainage.

## TREATMENT

Perirectal abscess is a true surgical emergency, and treatment with antibiotics alone is insufficient. Urgent drainage is always indicated in the emergency department, office, or operating room. The abscess should be opened as close to the anal verge as possible over the point of maximal fluctuance, and an adequate amount of skin should be removed to prevent premature closure. Digital lysis of loculations should be performed, and the cavity should be cultured, cleansed, irrigated, and packed for 24 hours. Antibiotics can be prescribed for cellulitis, fever, or leukocytosis or in immunosuppressed patients. Local wound care includes hot soaks and irrigation. Repacking is rarely necessary. Progression to a severe form of perineal sepsis (Fournier's gangrene, Meleney's synergistic gangrene, or necrotizing fasciitis) may occur with systemic signs such as fever, leukocytosis, and septic shock. Extensive débridement and fecal diversion may be necessary for treatment of complicated perineal sepsis.

Approximately 50% of perirectal abscesses will heal, but the remainder will form a chronic anorectal fistula tract. Non-inflammatory-bowel-disease-related anorectal fistulae always require surgery, but definitive repair should only be performed when the acute inflammatory process has subsided. A drain may be placed from the primary opening in the anal canal to the secondary opening on the perianal skin and tied to itself as a draining seton. This maintains the tract with adequate drainage until the inflammation subsides. Definitive repair consists of fistulotomy for simple anorectal fistulae in which the external anal sphincter is uninvolved or only minimally involved. The healing rate for fistulotomy is more than 90%, but it may take 2 months for the wound to completely granulate by secondary intention and epithelialize. A careful history for diarrheal illness should be elicited because anal fistula may be a manifestation of undiagnosed Crohn's disease. Complex anal fistula include tracts involving more than one-fourth (8 mm) of the external sphincter, rectovaginal fistulae, or fistulae occurring in Crohn's disease. Complex fistulae are treated with extra attention toward preservation of the anal sphincter. Several procedures are available, including suture repair with injection of fibrin sealant, endorectal advancement flap, anal fistula plug, or ligation of the intersphincteric fistula tract (LIFT procedure). The success rate of any given procedure is approximately 60%, and several procedures must sometimes be performed sequentially until healing occurs. Horseshoe perirectal abscess is a special circumstance in which a posterior anorectal fistula branches bilaterally into both ischiorectal fossae after penetrating the anococcygeal ligament. Treatment involves division of the anococcygeal ligament via a posterior midline counter-incision, as well as incision and drainage of both ischiorectal fossae with placement of Penrose drains communicating all three incisions (Hanley procedure).

# Anal Condyloma

## PRESENTATION AND DIAGNOSIS

Human papilloma virus (HPV) produces a variety of anorectal manifestations, including condyloma accuminata (venereal warts), verrucous carcinoma, and either low- or high-grade squamous intraepithelial neoplasia (LSIL or HSIL, respectively). HPV is sexually transmitted, and patients should be counseled regarding the contagious nature of the disease. Its subtypes 16 and 18 are associated with a high risk for development of squamous cell carcinoma. HPV can be asymptomatic or may produce verrucous anogenital lesions. These lesions can produce bleeding, pain, itching, or discharge and may involve the squamous epithelium of the anal canal, perianal skin, and genitalia. The verrucous growth occurs in response to the HPV virus, which resides in the dermis at the base of the wart. Anal condyloma may be biopsied for immunohistochemical subtyping to help assess future risk of malignancy.

## TREATMENT

Condyloma can be eradicated by using fulguration with electrocautery, laser, chemical, or cryogenic means. Recurrence is common and depends on the host's immune responsiveness. Local treatment with topical trichloroacetic acid (TCA) may be effective for small lesions, but it often requires repeated application. Topical imiquimod (Aldera) is an immunomodulatory drug effective in reducing the rate of recurrence by 25%. Patients with human immunodeficiency virus are especially at risk for development of HSIL and subsequent squamous cell carcinoma of the anus and require close surveillance with high-resolution anoscopy. These lesions may be identified by staining with acetic acid and Lugol's solution. Areas of HSIL are destroyed using infrared coagulation, laser vaporization, or electrocoagulation. All mass lesions of the anal canal and perianal skin should be suspected of harboring occult malignancy and should be biopsied.

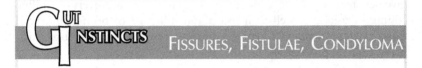

### FISSURES, FISTULAE, CONDYLOMA

1. Perirectal abscess is a surgical emergency and requires immediate incision and drainage.
2. Anorectal fistulae never heal without surgery. Although the failure rate for surgical repair is high, with persistence, successful closure with preservation of anal sphincter function is possible.
3. HPV infection can be a premalignant condition, especially in immunocompromised or human-immunodeficiency-virus-positive individuals, and requires intensive surveillance and preventive treatment for squamous intraepithelial lesions.
4. Always consider Crohn's disease in patients with anorectal disease (eg, skin tags, fissures, stenosis, or abscess or fistula formation). Always elicit a family history of inflammatory bowel disease or a personal history of a chronic diarrheal illness.
5. If an anal fissure is diagnosed, no further examination is usually necessary.

## Key Reference

1. Billingham RP, Isler JT, Kimmins MH, et al. The diagnosis and management of common anorectal problems. *Curr Probl Surg.* 2004;41(7):586-645.

# CHAPTER 31

# DIVERTICULAR DISEASE

Amy Lightner, MD and
James Yoo, MD, FACS, FASCRS

Although diverticulosis is extremely common, relatively few suscep-tible patients will actually develop symptoms. The majority of patients have asymptomatic diverticula found incidentally on imaging studies or endoscopy. Those who have symptoms typically present with either colonic bleeding secondary to diverticulosis or with diverticulitis. Diverticular disease may involve any part of the gastrointestinal (GI) tract, although the sigmoid colon is the most commonly affected segment. Colonic diverticula are false diverticula because only the mucosa and submucosa penetrate through the muscularis. While data are limited, it is postulated that high intraluminal pressure and a weak colonic wall lead to herniation at the sites of vessel penetration into the muscularis layer. A low-fiber diet, increased luminal pressure, abnormal colonic motility, defective muscular structure, defects in collagen con-sistency, and aging are associated with diverticula formation.

Although there are exceptions, diverticular disease primarily involves older patients in Western countries with low fiber intake. Before the age of 30, less than 2% of the population has diverticular disease whereas by the age of 85, an estimated 65% has the disease. Of interest, in Africa and Asia, the prevalence is a mere 0.2% and is typically right-sided, a notable difference from that seen in the United States.

Esrailian E. *Gut Instincts: A Clinician's Handbook of Digestive and Liver Diseases* (pp 211-216).
© 2012 Taylor & Francis Group

# Diverticulosis

## PRESENTATION

The overall evaluation and management of GI hemorrhage is discussed elsewhere in this text. Diverticular bleeding is the leading cause of brisk hematochezia, accounting for 30% to 50% of all lower GI bleeding. In patients with diverticulosis, roughly 15% will have bleeding secondary to their diverticular disease, and in 5%, the bleeding is severe. In 75% to 90% of patients, the bleeding will stop spontaneously. A reliable predictor of those who will stop bleeding is the number of units transfused. Of those transfused 4 or fewer units, the vast majority will stop bleeding spontaneously. Lower GI bleeding secondary to diverticulosis results when small blood vessels that are stretched over the dome of the diverticula rupture and bleed. Diverticular bleeding may be more common on the right, likely because the right colon has a thinner wall and the colonic diverticula have wider necks and domes, thereby creating a greater length over which vessels are exposed.

The patient typically presents with sudden, painless rectal bleeding accompanied by an urge to defecate. Patients usually do not have accompanying diverticulitis. The blood is typically bright red or maroon. Patients may be hemodynamically unstable depending on the rate of bleeding. On physical examination, patients do not complain of pain to abdominal palpation or rectal examination, but rectal examination may demonstrate bright red blood.

## DIAGNOSIS/MANAGEMENT

Refer to Chapter 23 for the evaluation and management of lower GI bleeding in general and for the role of colonoscopy. For diverticular bleeding, there are a few, often-utilized diagnostic modalities worth describing here. The Technetium (Tc)-99m labeled RBC nuclear medicine scan involves taking a few cc of blood from the patient, tagging the red blood cells extracorporeally with Tc and a tin compound, and then re-injecting the blood into the patient. Given the short half-life of Tc-99m, the patient has minimal radiation exposure as the study is completed. To identify active bleeding at a rate of 0.1 mL/min, the test has a sensitivity of 97%, specificity of 85%, and positive predictive value of 94%. Unfortunately, though highly sensitive, localization of active bleeding is inaccurate, requiring additional studies to confirm the location of the bleeding. If the scan is positive within the first few minutes, the likelihood of successful angiographic localization is increased significantly. In addition to localization, angiography can be useful for treatment with transcatheter embolization or the infusion of vasopressin. Operative intervention is necessary if the patient remains unstable despite aggressive resuscitation or for recurrent hemorrhage. A segmental resection can be performed if the area of bleeding has been localized. In patients with massive colonic bleeding without pre-operative localization, a subtotal colectomy with ileorectal anastomosis should be performed.

# Diverticulitis

## PRESENTATION

Diverticulitis refers to the inflammation that results from micro- or macroscopic perforation of the diverticulum. Most patients with diverticulosis will never develop diverticulitis, but publications describe incidence ranges generally from 10% to 25%. Microscopic perforation may fistulize, obstruct, or resolve spontaneously, whereas macroscopic perforation tends to cause peritonitis.

Patients typically complain of left lower quadrant abdominal pain that may radiate to the suprapubic area, left groin, or back; alteration in their bowel habits; fevers; chills; and urinary urgency. On physical examination, patients may have isolated tenderness at the left lower abdominal wall or an acute abdomen, depending on the severity of diverticulitis and potential complications. A tender mass in the lower left abdomen is suggestive of an abscess, and the patient may also be distended as a result of ileus from surrounding inflammation.

## DIAGNOSIS

If clinical suspicion is high, then the diagnosis can be based on history and physical examination alone, and antibiotics may be started early, even in the outpatient setting and if the symptoms are mild. A complete blood count (CBC) and computed tomography (CT) scan should be ordered to complete the diagnostic workup if emergency department or inpatient evaluation is warranted based on symptom severity. Leukocytosis may not be present in up to 60% of patients with diverticulitis. If indicated, CT reliably reveals the location of the infection, the extent of the inflammatory process, the presence and location of an abscess, any involvement with other organs by fistula or obstruction, and the potential to percutaneously drain any abscess detected.

## MANAGEMENT

The treatment of diverticulitis depends on the severity. Simple diverticulitis often can be treated with antibiotics on an outpatient basis, such as with ciprofloxacin 500 mg twice daily and metronidazole 500 mg, 3 times daily, for 10 to 14 days. If the patient has symptoms consistent with localized peritonitis, he or she should be admitted for broad-spectrum intravenous antibiotics (eg, ciprofloxacin and metronidazole). These patients' symptoms will usually improve within 48 hours, at which point they can be started on clear liquids and oral antibiotics until the fever and leukocytosis have resolved. There is a general consensus that operative intervention is not indicated for the first attack. However, there is some controversy in the surgical literature if an operation is indicated for patients who are young at the first attack or have multiple attacks.

Complicated diverticulitis is defined as diverticulitis with an associated abscess, phlegmon, or fistula (Figure 31-1). If a patient has an abscess, it should be drained percutaneously under CT or ultrasound guidance, unless it is small (<2 cm), and elective surgery should be considered. If a patient forms a fistula between the sigmoid colon and the skin, bladder, vagina, or small bowel, initial treatment is to control the infection and administer antibiotics followed by excision of the diseased colon to remove the fistula source. Perforation resulting in generalized peritonitis requires immediate operative intervention due to overwhelming infection.

In the immediate recovery period, a low-residue diet is important. After patients recover, they should remain on a high-fiber diet, and even use fiber supplements and stool softeners if needed, to prevent constipation. The lifetime risk of recurrence without surgery is estimated to be 25% after the first episode and 50% after the second attack. All should have a colonoscopy 6 weeks after the attack to rule out cancer, inflammatory bowel disease, or ischemia as the cause of the inflammatory mass.

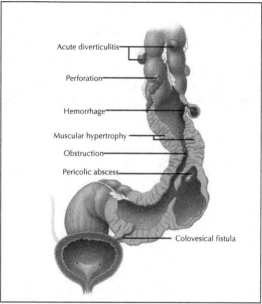

**Figure 31-1.** Acute diverticulitis and its complications including perforation, obstruction, abscess, and fistula formation. Reprinted with permission of Welch JP, Cohen JL. *ACS Surgery: Diverticulitis.* Decker Intellectual Properties; Philadelphia, PA: 2004.

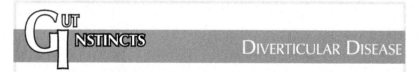

DIVERTICULAR DISEASE

1. Diverticular disease refers to diverticula of the colon, which are pseudodiverticula because the wall is composed of only the mucosa and submucosa.

2. Diverticular disease is primarily a Western disease and increases in prevalence with age.

3. The most important clinical complications of diverticular disease are bleeding and diverticulitis, but most people will never have either.

4. Diverticulitis represents micro- or macroscopic perforation of a diverticulum causing inflammation.

5. The hallmark of diverticular bleeding is painless rectal bleeding, and it is rare for diverticulitis to be present simultaneously.

# Key References

1. Fry RD, Mahmoud N, Maron DJ, Ross HM, Rombeau J. Colon and rectum. In: Townsend C, Beauchamp RD, Evers BM, Mattox K, eds. *Sabiston Textbook of Surgery: The Biological Basis of Modern Surgical Practice.* Philadelphia, PA: W.B. Saunders and Co; 2007:1364-1369.

2. Young-Fadok T, Pemberton JH. Clinical manifestations and diagnosis of colonic diverticular disease. In: UptoDate, Basow DS, ed. *UpToDate.* Waltham, MA; 2010.

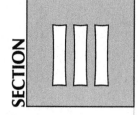

SECTION

III

# HEPATOLOGY

# ABNORMAL LIVER FUNCTION TESTS

Simon W. Beaven, MD, PhD

Elevated liver function tests (LFTs; ie, aspartate aminotransferase/ serum glutamic oxaloacetic transaminase [AST/SGOT], alanine aminotransferase/serum glutamic pyruvic transaminase [ALT/SPGT], total bilirubin, and alkaline phosphatase) are a common occurrence in clinical practice. Fortunately, the cause can usually be determined by a careful history and physical examination. With a sudden, marked elevation, or where no obvious risk factor is established, a liver biopsy should be considered. Initial evaluation emphasizes the chronicity (Figure 32-1) and absolute degree of elevation and pattern (Table 32-1). The first step should be to repeat the LFTs to be sure the elevations are real and persistent. Useful tests for establishing chronic liver disease include the platelet count, serum albumin, bilirubin, and coagulation parameters.

## Important Historical Features

### FATTY LIVER, OBESITY, AND INSULIN RESISTANCE

Metabolic syndrome is now recognized to include the hepatic correlate of insulin resistance: nonalcoholic fatty liver disease (NAFLD), covered in greater detail in Chapter 35. NAFLD is the most common cause of an abnormal ALT. Metabolic syndrome is defined by the presence of at least 2 to 3 of the following constellation of traits: obesity

Esrailian E. *Gut Instincts: A Clinician's Handbook of Digestive and Liver Diseases* (pp 219-226).
© 2012 Taylor & Francis Group

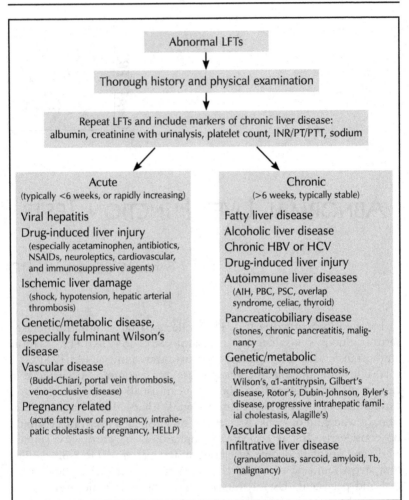

**Figure 32-1.** Initial evaluation emphasizing the chronicity. (LFT indicates liver function test; INR, international normalized ratio; PT, prothrombin time; PTT, partial thromboplastin time; NSAID, nonsteroidal anti-inflammatory drug; HBV, hepatitis B virus; HCV, hepatitis C virus; AIH, autoimmune hepatitis; PBC, primary biliary cirrhosis; PSC, primary sclerosing cholangitis; HELLP, hemolysis, elevated liver enzymes; Tb, tuberculosis)

(especially visceral abdominal obesity), diabetes/insulin resistance or glucose intolerance, dyslipidemia (both hypertriglyceridemia and low high-density lipoprotein levels), and hypertension.

| TABLE 32-1 | COMMON PATTERNS OF LIVER FUNCTION TEST ELEVATIONS | |
|---|---|---|
| **AST, ALT <500 U/L** | **AST, ALT >500 U/L** | |
| AST:ALT >2:1<br>• Consider alcoholic hepatitis, especially if pain, fever, hepatomegaly and AST, ALT <250<br><br>AST:ALT <2:1<br>• Most common pattern, but also the least specific. Any cause possible, most common are NAFLD/NASH, chronic viral hepatitis, alcoholic liver disease, and DILI. This is why history and physical are critical. | Consider acute liver failure (ALF) especially if AST or ALT >1000 U/L. If jaundice is present with either coagulopathy or mental status changes within 6 weeks of onset, seek consultation with a liver transplant center promptly. | |
| Common nonhepatic causes of elevated AST, ALT<br>• Celiac disease<br>• Thyroid disease<br>• Adrenal insufficiency<br>• Hemolysis<br>• Sepsis/shock<br>• Myocardial infarction<br>• Myopathy, including rhabdomyolysis<br>• Strenuous exercise<br><br>Isolated elevation alkaline phosphatase<br>• Nonhepatic<br>  o Heart failure<br>  o Pulmonary hypertension<br>  o Chronic renal failure<br>  o Lymphoma and malignancy (especially renal cell)<br>  o Bone disease<br>  o Pregnancy | • Acute viral hepatitis<br>  o Viral hepatitis A, B, C, D, E<br>  o HBV flare in an untreated, immunosuppressed patient<br>  o Cytomegalovirus, Epstein-Barr, influenza, adenovirus, parvo B19, herpes simplex (especially in pregnancy)<br>• DILI or toxin injury<br>  o Most common: Acetaminophen, NSAIDs, antibiotics, antifungals, antivirals, metformin, amlodarone, methotrexate, but essentially any Rx or OTC preparation, amanita mushroom, organophosphates<br>• Ischemic/shock liver<br>• Autoimmune hepatitis<br>• Wilson's disease<br><br>*(continued)* | |

## ALCOHOL USE

It is mandatory to conduct a thorough review of the pattern and duration of alcohol use. Alcoholic liver disease is covered in greater

| TABLE 32-1 | COMMON PATTERNS OF LIVER FUNCTION TEST ELEVATIONS (CONTINUED) |
|---|---|
| **AST, ALT <500 U/L** | **AST, ALT >500 U/L** |
| Isolated elevation alkaline phosphatase<br>• Hepatobiliary<br>  o Bile duct obstruction (stone/stricture)<br>  o PBC, PSC, or overlap syndrome<br>  o Cirrhosis<br>  o Chronic hepatitis<br>  o Hepatocellular carcinoma<br>  o Benign recurrent cholestasis<br>  o Vanishing bile duct sydrome (think meds)<br>  o Infiltrating disease (tumor, infection [Tb, fungal], granulomatous, sarcoid, amyloid) | Cholestatic predominant (primarily elevated bilirubin/alkaline phosphatase)<br>• Extrahepatic<br>  o Biliary tree disease: Gallstone, stricture, diverticulum, cholangiocarcinoma, ampullary cancer, metastatic lymph node compression at the porta hepatis<br>  o Pancreatic disease: Carcinoma, pseudocyst, chronic pancreatitis, IPMN<br>• Intrahepatic<br>  o PBC, PSC, or overlap syndrome<br>  o Diabetes<br>  o Sepsis<br>  o TPN/malnutrition<br>  o DILI (especially estrogens, androgens, steroids)<br>  o Infiltrating disease (tumor, infection [Tb, fungal], granulomatous, sarcoid, amyloid) |

AST indicates aspartate aminotransferase; ALT, alanine aminotransferase; PBC, primary biliary cirrhosis; PSC, primary sclerosing cholangitis; Tb, tuberculosis; IPMN, intrapapillary mucinous neoplasm; TPN, total parenteral nutrition; NAFLD, nonalcoholic fatty liver disease; NASH, nonalcoholic steatohepatitis; DILI, drug-induced liver injury; Rx, perscription drug; OTC, over the counter

detail in Chapter 36. Identification of problematic alcohol use, dependency, or abuse warrants further aggressive intervention because alcoholism is a treatable disease.

## VIRAL HEPATITIS

Risk factors for viral hepatitis (Chapters 33 and 34) should be investigated. The sudden onset of jaundice, dark urine, nausea, vomiting, fever, or abdominal pain should prompt consideration of acute viral hepatitis with appropriate serologic testing.

## DRUG-INDUCED LIVER INJURY

Drug-induced hepatotoxicity is an extremely common, but under-reported, occurrence. Thorough evaluation of prescription and non-prescription drug use is critical. Any drug (xenobiotic) is a potential hepatotoxin, and there should be a low threshold for stopping any/all medications if they are suspected of being the cause of elevated LFTs. Acetaminophen (APAP) toxicity is the leading cause of drug-induced liver failure in the United States (at least 40% of cases). Conversely, it is a common misconception that 3-hydroxy-3-methylglutaryl-coenzyme (HMG-CoA) reductase inhibitors lead to significant liver damage. Statins cause mild elevations of the AST/ALT without significant histologic disease or consequence. Periodic monitoring is prudent once an abnormality has been detected. Common nonprescription drug categories include over-the-counter (OTC), homeopathic, naturopathic, sleep aids, diet and weight loss, colon/liver cleansing preparations, and muscle/weight lifting supplements.

## AUTOIMMUNE DISEASE/IMMUNOLOGIC DYSFUNCTION

Autoimmune diseases of the liver include autoimmune hepatitis (AIH), primary biliary cirrhosis, and primary sclerosing cholangitis, and can present with mixed-pattern LFTs. Diagnosis should be made in consultation with a hepatologist. Chronic hepatitis C virus (HCV) infection is also associated with autoimmune antibodies. This is not a separate autoimmune disorder.

## MISCELLANEOUS CAUSES OF ABNORMAL LIVER FUNCTION TESTS

Overlooked causes include celiac disease and thyroid dysfunction. Muscle breakdown (myocardial infarction, myopathies, rhabdomyolysis) can lead to marked elevations of the AST/ALT. Cholestatic liver tests are also seen in pregnancy, malnutrition, and malabsorption. Infiltrative diseases such as amyloidosis, sarcoidosis, leukemia/lymphoma, and fungal/tuberculosis infections should be considered. Disorders of metabolism, including hereditary hemochromatosis, Wilson's disease, and alpha-1-antitrypsin (A1AT) deficiency should be considered with the appropriate clinical history, or if no other cause is apparent. Hemochromatosis is often mistakenly diagnosed based on abnormal iron studies in patients who have underlying alcoholism, HCV, and NAFLD, all of which can have secondary iron overload without an underlying genetic basis.

# Liver Function Tests

## ASPARTATE AMINOTRANSFERASE/ALANINE AMINOTRANSFERASE

These intracellular enzymes are involved in normal metabolic function, but spilled into the serum, they imply hepatocellular damage. Many clinicians equate them with markers of inflammation, but non-inflammatory causes of hepatocyte death (eg, apoptosis from drug-induced liver injury [DILI]) can lead to elevations. Normal values have been decreased considerably because reference populations previously included a large number of patients with NAFLD. Clinicians should use revised normal ALT levels cautiously as recent data suggest there is extensive short-term variation in AST/ALT levels. The importance of repeat testing cannot be over-emphasized in this situation. A single abnormal liver test value should not dictate whether a patient is committed to long-term therapy.

In alcoholic liver disease, the AST:ALT ratio is typically more than 2:1 because of the relative deficiency in vitamin $B_6$ (pyridoxal-5'-phosphate) among heavy drinkers. This deficiency decreases ALT serum activity more than AST and results in a perceived elevation of the AST:ALT ratio. In NAFLD, the AST:ALT is generally less than 1, and sometimes only the ALT is elevated. Alcoholic hepatitis almost never has AST/ALT levels greater than 250 U/L, so alternative diagnoses should be considered. Individuals with cirrhosis often have only slightly elevated levels of AST/ALT, and the tests may actually be normal (10% to 15%).

## BILIRUBIN

When evaluating bilirubin, it is important to determine both the direct (conjugated) and indirect (unconjugated) fractions. If more than 50% total bilirubin is in the unconjugated form, hemolysis should be suspected and consideration of nonhepatic causes of hyperbilirubinemia pursued. The most common causes of an isolated, unconjugated hyperbilirubinemia are hemolysis and Gilbert's disease (>50% unconjugated, total bilirubin approximately 2 to 9 mg/dL). Hyperbilirubinemia of sepsis is also a common entity in hospital practice. Conjugated hyperbilirubinemia is commonly caused by obstruction (gallstone, stricture, mass) or inflammation of the bile ducts, and an ultrasound is the first diagnostic test of choice.

## ALKALINE PHOSPHATASE

The liver fraction is found in the biliary epithelium and is, therefore, a measure of cholestatic dysfunction. Alkaline phosphatase (AP) isoforms are also produced in intestine, placenta, and bone. If there is no clear hepatic cause for elevation of this enzyme, AP isoforms can be useful for determining if the abnormality localizes to the liver or not. Congestive heart failure, renal dysfunction, infiltrating disease, and systemic malignancy can also lead to elevated AP. The gamma glutamyl transpeptidase (GGT) and 5'-nucleotidase are not routinely helpful. The GGT is mostly predictive of alcohol consumption but has a poor sensitivity/specificity for any particular liver disease. While almost all liver problems involve elevation of the liver function tests, a plummeting AP is a hallmark of acute Wilson's disease.

## Summary

The previous discussion emphasizes the history and physical examination in the evaluation of abnormal liver function tests. The judicious use of imaging can help support the diagnosis of biliary obstruction or chronic liver disease (cirrhosis) quite well, but imaging is less useful in the setting of acute liver failure. In most cases, liver biopsy should be reserved for staging known chronic liver disease (eg, prior to interferon/ribavirin therapy in chronic HCV) or for determining the underlying cause of abnormal LFTs when the history, physical, labs, and imaging do not point to a clear origin.

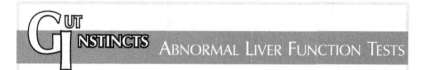

GUT INSTINCTS ABNORMAL LIVER FUNCTION TESTS

1. Cirrhosis is usually diagnosed with a thorough history and physical.
2. LFTs may be normal in cirrhosis. Thrombocytopenia is often the first laboratory abnormality. Low albumin and coagulopathy are also suggestive of cirrhosis.
3. Keys to diagnosing abnormal LFTs are chronicity, absolute degree of elevation, and pattern (hepatocellular versus cholestatic).
4. Usual causes of mildly abnormal LFTs: NAFLD, alcohol, chronic viral hepatitis, DILI, and autoimmune dysfunction.
5. When the cause is in doubt, referral to a hepatologist for biopsy is warranted.

# Key References

1. Pratt DS, Kaplan MM. Evaluation of abnormal liver-enzyme results in asymptomatic patients. *N Engl J Med*. 2000;342(17):1266-1271.
2. Lee WM. Drug-induced hepatotoxicity. *N Engl J Med*. 2003;349(5):474-485.
3. Lazo M, Selvin E, Clark JM. Brief communication: clinical implications of short-term variability in liver function test results. *Ann Intern Med*. 2008;148(5):348-352.

# CHAPTER 33

# HEPATITIS B

Vandana Khungar, MD, MSc and
Steven-Huy Han, MD, AGAF

More than 400 million people worldwide have chronic hepatitis B (CHB) infection. Up to 50% of the world's population has had hepatitis B virus (HBV) infection based on hepatitis B surface antibody (HBsAb) prevalence. HBV is endemic in countries that make up 45% of the world's population. In the United States, the prevalence of CHB infection is 0.1% to 0.2% (1.25 million), and the annual incidence of new infections is 200,000 to 300,000. HBV is transmitted mainly by perinatal, percutaneous, and sexual routes. In the United States, HBV is usually contracted via sexual or percutaneous routes; in Asia, perinatal transmission to infants from mothers with CHB occurs; and in sub-Saharan Africa, horizontal spread between young children occurs.

## Virologic Features and Pathogenesis

HBV is a partially double-stranded, partially single-stranded DNA virus (hepadnavirus Type 1) that replicates via reverse transcription, through a ribonucleic acid (RNA) intermediate, using a viral polymerase. Host immune responses against HBV, and not direct viral attack, are the principal determinants of hepatocellular injury. Patients with immunodeficiency who are infected with HBV often have mild acute liver injury, but high rates of chronic carriage.

Esrailian E. *Gut Instincts: A Clinician's Handbook
of Digestive and Liver Diseases* (pp 227-236).
© 2012 Taylor & Francis Group

# Hepatitis B Virus Mutants

Precore (PC) and basal core promoter (BCP) mutants constitute a naturally occurring variant of CHB termed *HBeAg-negative CHB*. This form of CHB is the predominant form in Europe but is now increasing in the United States. HBeAg-negative CHB is associated with lower levels of viral replication ($\leq 10^5$ virions/mL) than wild-type (HBeAg-positive) CHB ($\geq 10^6$ virions/mL). In HBeAg-negative CHB, because HBeAg seroconversion cannot be used as a treatment endpoint, the ideal duration of therapy remains undefined. Mutations occurring in the HBV polymerase are associated with resistance to antiviral agents such as lamivudine, adefovir, and telbivudine.

# Prevention

Recombinant hepatitis B vaccine is protective in more than 90% of normal adults and 100% of newborns. The immunogenicity of the vaccine is decreased in adults older than 40 years. In young, healthy adults, 2.5% to 5% do not acquire protective antibodies from the vaccine. Now, universal vaccination of all neonates and prepubertal teenagers is recommended. The HBV vaccine is also recommended in immunocompromised patients, hemodialysis patients, patients with co-existing chronic liver disease including chronic hepatitis C, health care workers, injection drug users, and those with high-risk sexual exposures.

# Clinical Findings and Diagnosis

During acute infection, HBV has an incubation period of 4 weeks to 6 months. Symptoms include fatigue, anorexia, and jaundice. Aminotransferase elevations are the most common laboratory abnormality. In 5% to 10% of cases, a serum sickness-like syndrome can develop. In children, acute hepatitis B can present as anicteric hepatitis with nonpruritic papular rash on the face, buttocks, and limbs.

Progression to chronic infection is defined as persistence of HBsAg for 6 or more months. Physical examination may be normal although hepatomegaly and splenomegaly may be noted in advanced disease. Laboratory testing indicates detectable HBeAg in HBeAg-positive patients and normal or abnormal aminotransferase, bilirubin, and globulin levels. Histology may be normal or show the presence of inflammation, varying degrees of fibrosis, or frank cirrhosis. Four distinct phases of CHB infection exist (immune tolerance, immune clearance, inactive carrier, and immune reactivation) characterized by the degree of alanine aminotransferase (ALT) elevation, quantitative HBV DNA level, and histology. In the immune tolerance phase, HBeAg is positive, DNA levels are elevated, and there is minimal liver injury. Flares often occur during the immune clearance phase, and DNA levels and ALT can fluctuate. In the inactive carrier phase, HBV DNA levels may be undetectable or low, and liver tests may appear normal as well. Finally, immune reactivation can occur with immunosuppression and can lead to significant inflammation and fibrosis. Patients often transition between phases. HBV diagnosis relies mainly on the presence of HBsAg. Acute and chronic infections are distinguished by other serologies (Table 33-1).

## Treatment

In fulminant hepatitis B, without intensive care unit (ICU) care, mortality approaches 80%. Protein intake is restricted, and oral lactulose or rifaximin is administered. Fluid and electrolyte balance are maintained, coagulation parameters monitored, broad-spectrum antibiotics started prophylactically, and treatment with oral nucleoside or nucleotide agents may be considered. Corticosteroid therapy can be harmful in fulminant hepatitis B. Patients are supported maximally until spontaneous recovery or until orthotopic liver transplantation (OLT).

In CHB, the goals are to suppress HBV replication and reduce liver injury. Endpoints include suppression of circulating HBV DNA; in HBeAg-positive chronic HBV, HBeAg seroconversion (loss of HBeAg and acquisition of anti-HBe); normalization of ALT levels; and improvement in liver histology. Successful therapy can delay progression to cirrhosis, decompensation, and the development of hepatocellular carcinoma (HCC). There are currently 7 therapies approved for the treatment of CHB (Table 33-2).

## Interferons (Interferon-α2b and Pegylated Interferon-α2a)

Interferon-α (IFNα)-2b was the first antiviral approved for hepatitis B. The strongest predictor of response to IFNα in HBeAg-positive patients is a high pretreatment ALT level. In patients with HBeAg-positive disease, the course is 16 to 24 weeks. Other favorable factors are high histologic activity index, low HBV DNA level, and HBV genotypes A and B. In HBeAg-negative patients, longer courses of IFNα are necessary (12 to 18 months). IFNα is absolutely contraindicated in patients with decompensated cirrhosis because it can precipitate hepatic failure or life-threatening infection. Other contraindications include immune suppression or autoimmune disease and severe, uncontrolled psychiatric

## HEPATITIS B SEROLOGIES

**TABLE 33-1**

| HBsAg | HBeAg | IgM anti-HBc | IgG anti-HBc | Anti-HBs | Anti-HBe | HBV DNA | Interpretation |
|---|---|---|---|---|---|---|---|
| | | | | | | | Susceptible |
| | | | + | + | | | Immune due to natural infection |
| | | | | + | | | Immune due to hepatitis B vaccination |
| + | + | | | | | +++ | Early acute infection |
| | | + | | | | + | Window phase |
| | | | + | + | + | ± | Recovery phase |
| + | + | | + | | | +++ | Chronic replicative phase |
| + | | | + | | + | ± | Chronic low nonreplicative phase |
| + | ± | + | + | | | + | Flare of chronic HBV |
| + | | | + | | + | ++ | Precore/core promoter mutants |
| | | | + | | | | Four possibilities: 1. Resolved infection 2. False-positive anti-HBc, so susceptible 3. Low level chronic infection 4. Resolving acute infection |

HBsAg indicates hepatitis B surface antigen; HBeAg, hepatitis B e antigen; IgM, immunoglobulin M; IgG, immunoglobulin G; anti-HBc, anti-hepatitis B core; Anti-HBs, anti-hepatitis B surface; Anti-HBe, anti-hepatitis B "e"; HBV DNA, hepatitis B virus DNA

| Table 33-2 | Federal Drug Administration Approved Oral Antivirals for Chronic Hepatitis B | | | | |
|---|---|---|---|---|---|
| | **Lamivudine** | **Adefovir** | **Entecavir** | **Telbivudine** | **Tenofovir** |
| Year of approval | 1998 | 2002 | 2005 | 2006 | 2008 |
| Abbreviation | LAM | ADV | ETV | TBV | TNV |
| Mechanism of action | Blocks HBV reverse transcriptase | Blocks HBV reverse transcriptase | Inhibits HBV DNA polymerase | Inhibits HBV DNA polymerase | Inhibits HBV DNA polymerase |
| Clearance | Renal | Renal | Renal | Renal | Renal |
| Dose | 100 mg/day | 10 mg/day | 0.5 mg/day | 600 mg/day | 300 mg/day |
| Renal and dialysis adjusted dose | 50 mg/day | 10 mg/day | 0.25 mg/day or 0.5 mg every other day | 600 mg every other day | 300 mg every other day |
| Common side effects | Occasional myopathy, neuropathy, pancreatitis | Nephrotoxicity, pancreatitis | Negligible | Myopathy | Nephrotoxicity |
| Pregnancy category | C | C | C | B | B |
| HBV DNA undetectability rates | 40% to 44% | 21% | 67% | 60% | 76% |
| HBeAg seroconversion rates | 16% to 21% | 12% | 21% | 22% | 21% |
| LAM indicates lamivudine; ADV, adefovir; ETV, entecavir; TBV, telbivudine; TNV, tenofovir; HBV, hepatitis B virus; HBeAg, hepatitis B "e" antigen | | | | | |

disease, or depression. Side effects include flu-like symptoms, marrow suppression, anxiety, depression, and autoimmune disorders. IFNα is accompanied by a flare in ALT in 30% to 40% of patients, which is usually predictive of a favorable response but, in patients with advanced cirrhosis, can precipitate decompensation.

IFNα has largely been replaced by long-acting, once-weekly pegylated interferon (PEG-IFN). PEG-IFNs are larger molecular weight interferon molecules with decreased renal clearance and increased half-life. PEG IFNα2a is the only pegylated interferon approved for chronic HBV in the United States. It is generally used for 48 weeks at a dose of 180 mcg weekly. The side effect profile is similar to standard interferon.

# Nucleos(t)ide Analogs

The oral nucleos(t)ide drugs are administered once daily. These newer drugs are potent in suppressing HBV replication with efficacy rates and HBeAg seroconversion rates summarized in Table 33-2. Endpoints with oral antiviral therapy are usually HBeAg serconversion in HBeAg-positive patients and undetectable HBV DNA in HBeAg-negative patients. However, long-term or indefinite therapy is usually required in HBeAg-negative patients due to the high relapse rates (return of elevated HBV DNA and ALT levels) following antiviral drug discontinuation. Resistance is the major concern with some oral antivirals, although entecavir and tenofovir have very low resistance rates.

## LAMIVUDINE

Lamivudine is an oral nucleoside analog originally used for the treatment of HIV. Lamivudine is safe to use in cirrhosis or hepatic decompensation. With monotherapy, genotypic resistance is noted in 14% to 32% of patients after the first year and increases to 60% to 70% after 5 years. The most prevalent mutation is a substitution of methionine for valine or isoleucine in the tyrosine-methionine aspartate-aspartate (YMDD) motif of the HBV DNA polymerase. Long duration of treatment, high pretreatment serum HBV DNA, and high levels of residual virus after initiation of treatment are associated with resistance. Lamivudine resistance is detected by virologic breakthrough, then biochemical breakthrough. If there is confirmed resistance, patients should receive rescue therapy with tenofovir or adefovir. The new drug is added to lamivudine; sequential monotherapy is discouraged due to the risk of multidrug resistance. Lamivudine is no longer recommended as first-line treatment for CHB due to its high resistance rates.

## ADEFOVIR

Adefovir is a nucleotide effective against wild-type and lamivudine-resistant HBV. It produces a histologic response in 53% of HBeAg-positive patients after 48 weeks, HBeAg seroconversion in 12%, normalization of ALT levels in 48%, and $3.5 \log_{10}$ copies/mL decrease in HBV DNA. Despite this success, up to 30% of patients with no prior nucleotide treatment will have a primary nonresponse, and other medications must be used. Adefovir has also been effective in OLT recipients, HIV-HBV coinfected patients, and lamivudine-resistant HBV.

## TELBIVUDINE

Telbivudine is more potent than lamivudine. In HBeAg-positive patients, DNA was undetectable in 54% after 2 years. Although rates of virologic and biochemical improvement are higher with telbivudine than lamivudine, no difference was seen in the rate of HBeAg seroconversion. In HBeAg-negative patients, telbivudine was superior to lamivudine. A high degree of resistance (21.6% of HBeAg-positive patients after 2 years, 8.6% of HBeAg-negative patients after 2 years) exists. Telbivudine selects for tyrosine-methionine-aspartate-aspartate (YMDD) mutations, so there is cross-resistance with lamivudine. Telbivudine has also not been recommended as first-line monotherapy for HBV infection.

## ENTECAVIR

Entecavir is a newer nucleoside analog drug that is more potent than lamivudine and adefovir. Entecavir is administered at a dose of 0.5 mg daily for treatment-naïve patients and 1.0 mg for lamivudine-resistant patients. Entecavir has very little resistance (less than 1% of treatment-naïve patients through year 5 of treatment). In lamivudine-resistant patients, entecavir resistance is up to 43% at 4 years. It is a good first-line treatment for previously untreated patients but is not recommended for treatment of lamivudine-resistant patients. In HBeAg-positive patients, after 48 weeks of treatment, entecavir has excellent histologic (72%), virologic (67% undetectable HBV RNA), and biochemical (68% with normal ALT) response. Of the 21% of patients who underwent seroconversion during the first year and stopped treatment at 48 weeks, 70% remained HBeAg negative. In HBeAg-negative patients, excellent histologic, virologic, and biochemical improvement is also seen, but relapse is noted if treatment is stopped after 1 year.

## TENOFOVIR

Tenofovir is very similar to, but more potent than, adefovir for treatment and resistance profiles. It is particularly useful in co-infected patients. To date, no resistance to tenofovir has been found in CHB patients after 3 years of therapy.

# Summary

Most adults (95% to 99%) recover completely from acute HBV infection. The risk of developing chronic HBV is related to the age of acquisition (90% in newborns, 50% in young children, 50% in immunocompromised adults, and 1% to 5% in immunocompetent adults). Patients with CHB usually fall into 1 of 4 different phases of infection, including immune tolerance, immune clearance, inactive, or reactivation. Hepatitis B accounts for half of fulminant viral hepatitis cases. Patients with CHB, whether HBeAg positive or negative, can develop cirrhosis, hepatic decompensation, and HCC. Those with high serum HBV DNA levels (>$10^5$ virions/mL) are more likely to have these complications. Cirrhosis is present in 70% to 80% of HBV-related HCC. Hepatocellular carcinoma is the leading cause of cancer-related death in regions where HBV is endemic. Chronic hepatitis B is unique in that 20% to 30% of patients with HCC do not have underlying cirrhosis. Alfa fetoprotein and liver ultrasound are recommended for HCC surveillance, but have not been shown to reduce mortality from HCC in CHB.

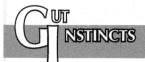

HEPATITIS B

1. Universal hepatitis B vaccination is recommended in all neonates, prepubertal teenagers, immunocompromised patients, hemodialysis patients, patients with co-existing chronic liver disease, health care workers, injection drug users, and those with high-risk sexual exposures.
2. There are 4 different phases of hepatitis B infection: immune tolerance, immune clearance, inactive, or reactivation.
3. Interferon is contraindicated in patients with decompensated cirrhosis.
4. Lamivudine has high resistance rates and is no longer recommended as first-line treatment for chronic hepatitis B.
5. Entecavir and tenofovir have low resistance rates, adefovir is useful in HIV-HBV co-infected patients, and telbivudine has high resistance rates.

## Key References

1. Lok AS. Chronic hepatitis B. Update 2009. *Hepatology.* 2009;50(3):661-662.
2. European Association for the Study of the Liver. EASL clinical practice guidelines: management of chronic hepatitis B. *J Hepatology.* 2009;50(2):227-242.
3. Dienstag JL. Hepatitis B virus infection. *N Engl J Med.* 2008;359(14): 1486-1500.

# HEPATITIS C

Ke-Qin Hu, MD

Hepatitis C virus (HCV) infection is a major public health problem. Approximately 180 million people are infected by HCV worldwide. In the United States, the prevalence of HCV infection was 1.6%, or 4.1 million people, and 80% of them have ongoing infection. HCV-cirrhosis is the principal cause of death from liver disease and the leading indication for liver transplantation in the United States.

Injection drug use is currently the primary risk for HCV transmission in the United States. Thus, all individuals who use or have used illicit injection drugs should be tested for HCV infection. Patients who have received a blood or blood-component transfusion or an organ transplant before 1992, and hemophiliacs receiving blood products before 1987, should be screened for HCV infection. Similarly, those with unexplained elevations of elevated liver enzymes or those ever on hemodialysis, children born to HCV-infected mothers, or those with human immunodeficiency virus (HIV) infection should be tested. Other risks include exposure to an infected sexual partner, multiple sexual partners, and exposure of health care workers to HCV-contaminated body fluid.

To prevent further HCV transmission, counseling should be provided to all infected patients about a healthy lifestyle, recommending notifying their current partners of their HCV status, and discussing the risk of sexual transmission, which is from 1% to 5% among monogamous sexual partners of index HCV cases.

Esrailian E. *Gut Instincts: A Clinician's Handbook of Digestive and Liver Diseases* (pp 237-244).

# Diagnostic Testing for Hepatitis C Virus Infection

## HEPATITIS C VIRUS-RELATED LABORATORY TESTS

The third generation of anti-HCV test is highly sensitive and specific, and it is the recommended serologic screening test. The HCV virologic tests include HCV ribonucleic acid (RNA) and genotyping. A sensitive quantitative HCV RNA polymerase chain reaction (PCR) test is recommended to confirm HCV infection and determine response to HCV treatment. Although there may be more, 6 different HCV genotypes (GT) are commonly determined by genotyping.

## LIVER BIOPSY

Liver biopsy has been widely regarded as the gold standard to assess liver disease status, although it may carry risks (eg, pain, bleeding), may require special expertise for interpreting the histopathology, and may be subject to sampling error. It provides valuable information on grade of the liver injury, stage of fibrosis, assessing chronic hepatitis C (CHC) progression, and is helpful in therapy decision making.

# Making the Diagnosis

Anti-HCV is a standard screen test, but it cannot differentiate ongoing HCV infection with past infection. Thus, an HCV RNA test, preferably a sensitive quantitative PCR test, should be performed in all individuals who test positive for anti-HCV to further confirm the diagnosis of ongoing HCV infection. Those who are positive for anti-HCV, but negative for HCV RNA (again confirmed by a repeated sensitive HCV RNA test), meet the criteria of past HCV infection.

HCV infection can be further divided into acute or chronic. After acute exposure, HCV RNA is usually detected in serum before antibody; HCV RNA can be identified as early as 2 weeks following exposure, whereas anti-HCV is generally not detectable before 8 to 12 weeks. These 2 markers of HCV infection may be present in varying per mutations, requiring careful analysis for interpretation. Chronic HCV infection is defined as the infection that persists for more than 6 months. The differentiation of acute from chronic HCV infection depends on the clinical presentation, namely the presence of the related symptoms and signs and a prior history of alanine aminotransferase (ALT) elevation and its duration.

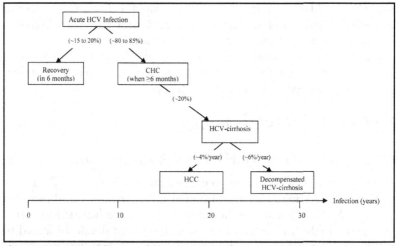

**Figure 34-1.** Natural history of chronic HCV infection. (HCV indicates hepatitis C virus; CHC, chronic hepatitis C; HCC, hepatocellular carcinoma)

Some patients may present with a positive test for anti-HCV, but a negative test for HCV RNA. This may represent acute HCV infection with transient clearance of HCV RNA, a false-positive anti-HCV or negative HCV RNA result or, more commonly, recovery from HCV infection. Retesting for HCV RNA in 4 to 6 months is recommended to confirm the resolution of HCV infection. The reverse scenario (ie, a negative anti-HCV test, but a positive test for HCV RNA) may indicate an early stage of acute infection prior to the development of antibody, or chronic infection in immunocompromised status. Alternatively, it may represent a false-positive HCV RNA result. These individuals should undergo retesting for anti-HCV and HCV RNA in 4 to 6 months to further address the issue.

## Natural History

Serum ALT can be elevated, and HCV RNA could be detectable within 7 to 10 days after initial exposure, but only approximately 20% of patients become symptomatic after an acute HCV infection. As shown in Figure 34-1, 80% to 85% of acute HCV infection will become chronic (persistent HCV RNA for ≥6 months). The reported risk for developing cirrhosis in these patients is approximately 20% after 2 to 3 decades of infection, but it varies depending on the patients studied. HCV-cirrhosis carries increased risk (~2% to 4% per year) for hepatocellular carcinoma (HCC). Thus, these patients should regularly undergo HCC surveillance. Many factors have been associated with CHC progression and risk for cirrhosis. These can be further classified as host-related (eg, age of infection and presentation, race, gender), lifestyle- or environment-related (eg, alcohol use), and virology-related (eg, duration of infection, HCV load and genotypes) factors. Effective HCV treatment has been associated with improved outcomes.

# Hepatitis C Virus Therapy

## INDICATION AND GOALS OF HEPATITIS C VIRUS TREATMENT

HCV treatment should be considered in all HCV-infected patients with active liver injury and increased risk for cirrhosis (ie, those with elevated ALT and/or histological evidence of active hepatic inflammation and/or advanced stage of fibrosis). Treatment should be aimed to effectively suppress HCV replication, thereby reducing liver injury and preventing progression to cirrhosis and its complications.

## PATTERNS OF TREATMENT RESPONSE

End of treatment response (ETR) is defined as undetectable HCV RNA at the end of an HCV treatment. Sustained virologic response (SVR) is defined as undetectable HCV RNA by a sensitive HCV RNA PCR assay 24 weeks after an HCV treatment is discontinued. Studies have demonstrated that once achieving SVR, the response associated with good long-term outcomes is usually durable. Thus, SVR should be considered the best surrogate of the goal and/or end point for HCV treatment. Rapid virologic response (RVR) is defined as undetectable HCV RNA 4 weeks after an HCV treatment is initiated and is highly predictive to SVR independent of HCV genotype and the treatment regimen. Patients who achieve an RVR may be able to shorten the duration of treatment. In contrast, because of a poor negative predictive value, the absence of an RVR should not be used for discontinuing HCV treatment. Complete early virologic response (EVR) is defined as undetectable HCV RNA 12 weeks after an HCV treatment is initiated. The absence of an EVR is the most important way to identify nonresponders. Thus, patients who do not have an EVR can discontinue HCV therapy early without compromising their chance to achieve an SVR. Nonresponder is defined as unable to achieve undetectable HCV RNA at the end of an HCV treatment. Relapser is defined as redetectable HCV RNA in someone who achieved ETR virologic response.

## TREATMENT REGIMENS

The currently recommended therapy of CHC is the combination of PEG-IFN-α, including α-2a and α-2b, and ribavirin (RBV), that was demonstrated to be superior to the standard interferon (IFN)-α and RBV. The original recommended dose of PEG-IFN-α-2b was 1.5 µg/kg/week with a fixed dose of RBV, 800 mg/day. A subsequent community-based study demonstrated that body weight-based RBV (800 to 1400/day) was more effective, especially in those with HCV GT-1 infection. A PEG-IFN-α-2a is administered at a fixed dose of 180 µg/week together with RBV, 1000 (for a body weight of less than 75 kg) to 1200 mg (for a body weight of 75 kg or more) daily. The treatment duration varies with HCV GT. For those with HCV GT-2 or -3 infection, the recommended treatment duration is 24 weeks; whereas, the duration for those with other HCV GT infection is typically 48 weeks. It should be noted that IFN or PEG-IFN is contraindicated in those with allergic reaction for these drugs, uncontrolled depression, or autoimmune disorders. Ribavirin is contraindicated for those who are or plan to be pregnant and those with renal insufficiency.

# Factors Associated With Hepatitis C Virus Treatment Response

Many host, viral, and other factors may influence the outcome of HCV treatment (ie, SVR rates). Understanding these will help in making treatment decisions. Viral factors include HCV GT and baseline viral count. HCV GT-2 and GT-3 respond to treatment best, but HCV GT-1 is most resistant to HCV treatment. The recent finding that the genetic polymorphisms of interleukin-28B (IL28B) locus are highly associated with HCV treatment response indicates the importance of the host genetic features contributing to response level. Other host factors, including race, age, and gender, have been well associated with HCV treatment response. Factors, such as CHC disease stage, co-infection with hepatitis B virus, HIV, and HCV treatment regimens, have also been associated with HCV treatment response.

# Pre-Treatment Assessment and Monitoring During/After Hepatitis C Virus Treatment

Besides the indication for HCV treatment, all patients should undergo a thorough assessment for aforementioned contraindications to IFN and RBV treatment. It is advisable to assess the risk of underlying coronary heart disease, to control pre-existing medical problems, such as

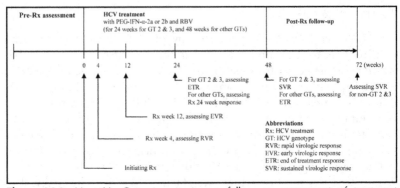

**Figure 34-2.** Hepatitis C treatment course, follow-up, assessment of treatment response when using peginterferon and ribavirin regimens. (RBV indicates ribavirin; PEG-IFN, peginterferon)

uncontrolled diabetes and hypertension, and to prescreen all candidates for symptoms of depression prior to initiating HCV therapy.

Patients should be monitored during therapy to assess the response to treatment and for the occurrence of side effects. A reasonable schedule would be monthly visits during the first 12 weeks of treatment followed by visits at 8- to 12-week intervals thereafter until the end of therapy. At each visit, the patient should be questioned regarding the presence of side effects and depression and provided with support regarding adherence to the treatment. Laboratory monitoring should include measurement of the complete blood count, serum creatinine and ALT levels, and HCV RNA by a sensitive assay at weeks 4, 12, and 24; 4- to 12-week intervals thereafter; at the end of treatment; and 24 weeks after stopping treatment (Figure 34-2). Thyroid function should be monitored every 12 weeks while on treatment.

# Hepatitis C Virus Retreatment and the New Hepatitis C Virus Therapy Under Development

Approximately 20% to 60% of patients treated with PEG-IFN and RBV will not achieve an SVR, due to nonresponse, virological breakthrough, or relapse. Planning retreatment will depend on the detailed history of and the pattern of the response to prior HCV treatment. Both prolonged course and higher dose regimens have been tested, but the results are disappointing, especially those null nonresponders. For more information on HCV retreatment, refer to the references.

Introduction of HCV specifically target antiviral therapy (STAT-C), or direct-acting antiviral (DAA) therapy represents a novel approach to HCV treatment. For instance, recent phase 3 clinical trials have demonstrated that the addition of a protease inhibitor (ie, boceprevir and telaprevir) to the current standard of care (SOC) HCV treatment regimens, PEG-IFN plus RBV, could significantly increase SVR rates from approximately 40% (PEG-IFN plus RBV) to approximately 60-75% in both naïve and prior treatment failure patients with HCV genotype 1 infection. These novel treatment regimens will revolutionize our SOC in HCV treatment soon after US Food and Drug Administration approval. However, evidence-based utilization of response guided therapy, good knowledge and experience in managing treatment-related adverse effects, careful patient follow up and constant support will be essential for optimizing the effects of these new HCV treatment regimens.

Several other DAA agents with different HCV targeting sites are being developed and the early data seem promising. Once confirmed by the clinical trials, these new treatment regimens will provide us with more effective options in managing CHC.

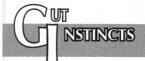

### HEPATITIS C

1. CHC is one of the most common chronic liver diseases among individuals in the United States. Cirrhosis and hepatocellular carcinoma can be the long-term complication in some of these patients.

2. Individuals who carry risks for HCV infection, such as those who use or have used illicit injection drugs or received blood/blood product transfusions before 1992, should undergo HCV screening.

3. Currently used anti-HCV test is a sensitive and specific test to screen for HCV infection, and a sensitive HCV ribonucleic acid polymerase chain reaction test should be used to confirm HCV infection.

4. Pegylated interferon in combination with ribavirin is currently the standard treatment for CHC; the sustained response rate is 40% to 80% depending on many virologic, host, and treatment factors.

5. Introduction of HCV DAA therapy, such as HCV protease inhibitors (ie, boceprevir and telaprevir), significantly increases SVR rates in both naïve and prior treatment failure patients with HCV GT-1 infection.

# Key References

1. Bialek SR, Terrault N. The change in epidemiology and natural history of hepatitis C virus infection. *Clin Liv Dis.* 2006;10(4):697-715.
2. Ghany MG, Strader DB, Thomas DL, Leonard B, Seeff LB. Diagnosis, management, and treatment of hepatitis C: an update. *Hepatology.* 2009;49(4): 1335-1374.
3. Asselah T, Marcellin P. Newdirect-acting antivirals' combination for the treatment of chronic hepatitis C. *Liver Int.* 2011;(31 Suppl 1):68-77.

# NONALCOHOLIC FATTY LIVER DISEASE

Michel H. Mendler, MD, MS

Nonalcoholic fatty liver disease (NAFLD) is the most prevalent chronic liver disease in the United States. It is associated with insulin resistance and, in most instances, is a benign condition. However, it can progress to nonalcoholic steatohepatitis (NASH), cirrhosis, and even hepatocellular carcinoma (HCC).

## Definition and Natural History

Secondary fatty liver disease is due to either liver diseases, such as alcoholic liver disease, viral hepatitis, autoimmune hepatitis, and Wilson's disease, or nonhepatic processes, such as drug-induced steatosis (amiodarone), jejunal bypass, protein malnutrition, or rare lipoprotein deficiencies. Primary fatty liver disease is due to obesity, diabetes mellitus Type 2 (DM2), and hyperlipidemia. It can present as a spectrum of pathology mimicking that of alcoholic liver disease (ALD). The basic form of NAFLD consists of macrovesicular steatosis. The more progressive form of NASH presents with the same features of acute alcoholic hepatitis, but most often to a lesser degree, including steatosis, a mixed lobular infiltrate predominating in neutrophils, hepatoctye ballooning, necrosis and Mallory bodies, and sinusoidal fibrosis. Ultimately, NASH can progress to cirrhosis. In the later stages of cirrhosis, the steatosis and inflammation may even be absent. While NAFLD presents with cirrhosis typically only after many years of progression, significant numbers of pediatric cases arising in teenagers are increasingly being reported due

Esrailian E. *Gut Instincts: A Clinician's Handbook of Digestive and Liver Diseases* (pp 245-250).
© 2012 Taylor & Francis Group

to the childhood obesity epidemic. Some patients, in particular White patients, can present with mild to moderate iron deposition (Perl's stain) in sinusoidal cells (Kupffer cells) in relation to the hepatic iron overload syndrome (IR-HIO). Several pathological grading and scoring systems exist for NAFLD but, in clinical practice, most pathologists report results as steatosis, NASH, or cirrhosis.

## Pathophysiology

The current hypothesis is that NAFLD progresses via a "multiple hit" process. Evidence suggests that insulin resistance is the principle first hit. A fat- and carbohydrate-laden high-calorie diet and lack of aerobic physical activity lead to increased levels of circulating insulin, ultimately insulin resistance, and an alteration of trygliceride metabolism. This sequence results in elevated abdominal fat deposition and other components of the metabolic syndrome (ie, obesity, arterial hypertension, hyperlipidemia). The second hit leading to NASH is less understood, and theories range from direct toxic effects of lipid peroxidation to recruitment of pro-inflammatory pathways. The third hit may well be time.

## Epidemiology

The prevalence of NAFLD is inexorably increasing in developed countries and mirrors the growing worldwide epidemic of obesity. The highest prevalence is found in the United States, which boasts the highest rate of adult obesity (body mass index [BMI] higher than 30) approaching 35% of the population. Current estimates are that at least 20% of the US adult population has NAFLD. The NASH prevalence estimates are less precise and are thought to be between 2% to 4%. The prevalence of cirrhosis due to NAFLD is difficult to estimate, but it is an ever-increasing indication for liver transplantation. There is also higher prevalence in Hispanic populations in the United States.

## Clinical Presentation

NAFLD is typically an incidental diagnosis upon the fortuitous finding of mildly elevated transaminases and/or a fatty liver on abdominal imaging. The most frequent findings are those of metabolic syndrome/ insulin resistance, including abdominal obesity ("pot belly" or "apple obesity"), arterial hypertension, and acathosis nigricans. Transaminases can be normal or mildly to moderately elevated (up to 8 to 10 times the upper normal limit). Typically, alanine aminotranferase (ALT) elevations are greater than aspartate aminotransferase (AST). Alkaline phosphatase can be mildly elevated, and gamma-glutamyl transferase can be strongly increased, mimicking alcoholic liver disease. Triglycerides, total cholesterol, low-density lipoproteins, fasting blood glucose, and hemoglobin A1c may be elevated. Ferritin may be up to 5 to 7 times upper normal limit with normal transferrin levels and saturation, and the absence of C282Y HFE homozygosity, suggesting IR-HIO (Figure 35-1).

## Diagnosis in Clinical Practice

Alcoholic liver disease should be excluded by history. Consumption of 20 g/d in women or 40 g/d in men for at least 1 year is associated with an odds ration of 2 for ALD; AST level greater than ALT is highly suspicious for ALD. If ALD is suspected or denied, an elevated level of serum carbohydrate-deficient transferrin (CDT) is a good screen for chronic alcohol abuse. All patients should be screened for hepatitis C virus (HCV)/hepatitis B virus (HBV). Of note, HCV genotype 3 can be associated with steatosis even in the absence of a metabolic syndrome. Ceruloplasmin levels testing for Wilson's disease should be obtained in patients younger than age 30. Autoimmune markers (antibodies to nuclei and smooth muscle antibodies) should be obtained, but caution should be used not to overinterpret low titers because they are present in at least 20% of the general population (see Figure 35-1).

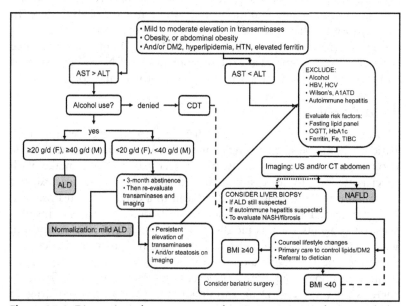

**Figure 35-1.** Diagnosis and management of NAFLD. (OGTT indicates oral glucose tolerance test; CT, computed tomography; HTN, hypertension)

The suspicion of NAFLD is confirmed by a negative workup and positive finding of steatosis on imaging. Ultrasound is the most frequently used imaging modality, demonstrating an enlarged diffuse echogenic ("brilliant") parenchyma relative to the kidney, a smooth edge, and a well-demarcated hepatic vasculature. Unfortunately, obesity decreases the sensitivity of ultrasound due to the reflection of ultrasound waves by abdominal adipose tissue. Computed tomography (CT) can show a diffusely hypodense liver of at least 10 Hounsfield units relative to the spleen. In 5% to 10% of cases, the distribution of steatosis is irregular due to portal perfusion variations, more prominent in the right than the left lobe, or presenting with irregular "drop-out" zones leading to the erroneous impression of a liver mass.

A liver biopsy is typically not indicated, unless the picture is not clear. Biopsy should be performed if there are significant risks for autoimmune hepatitis, such as in women with elevated serum globulins and quantitative immunoglobulin G, strongly positive autoimmune markers, and a history of another autoimmune disease (Hashimoto's thyroiditis being the most common). Suspicion of ALD in the face of strong denial of alcohol use can also be an indication for a liver biopsy but, as previously mentioned, NAFLD and ALD share the same features. In ALD, they are typically accentuated, and a positive CDT in this setting can be helpful in differentiating the two. If there is only moderate alcohol use, then a good test is to ask the patient to stop all alcohol consumption and to check transaminases and ultrasound after 3 months of abstinence. In straightforward diagnoses of NAFLD, a liver biopsy does have the benefit of grading and staging the severity of NAFLD but will not change management. In some cases, the demonstration of NASH and fibrosis can increase patient motivation to follow treatment and compliance.

## Treatment

The treatment is simple, yet difficult, to achieve—weight loss. Patients should be strongly encouraged to make common-sense lifestyle choices, such as aerobic exercise and a decrease in calorie intake, with special attention to decreasing carbohydrates and fats. Regular exercise alone, even without weight loss, can lead to a decrease in steatosis and inflammation. There have been several well-conducted trials of insulin-sensitizing agents such as pioglitazone, rosiglitazone, and metformin, with and without antioxidants such as vitamin E, or with S-adenosyl-L-methionine or betaine alone. They have shown some improvements in liver histology, but the positive changes are short lived. To date, there is no Food and Drug Administration (FDA)-approved drug to treat NAFLD. Clinicians should be reassured regarding using statins to control lipids in these patients. They can elevate transaminases moderately, but this effect is due to changes in the metabolism of these enzymes and not due to drug-induced hepatitis. Once on statins, persistent elevations in enzymes can cloud their interpretation, but the benefit of controlling lipids in preventing cardiovascular disease far outweighs this inconvenience. Control of DM2 should be optimized. For the morbidly obese (BMI >40) who are not cirrhotic, bariatric surgery is a valuable option leading to significant improvements in NAFLD and other parameters of insulin resistance. Lastly, patients should be counseled to not drink alcohol (see Figure 35-1).

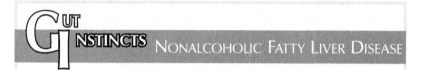

1. NAFLD is the most prevalent chronic liver disease in the United States.
2. NAFLD is most often benign, but it can progress to nonalcoholic steatohepatitis and cirrhosis and is becoming a major indication for liver transplantation. It is increasing being associated with other chronic liver disease, such as HCV.
3. Typical presentation is one of mildly elevated transaminases, with alanine aminotransferase greater than aspartate aminotransferase, in association with elements of insulin resistance: obesity and/or abdominal obesity, prediabetes or diabetes mellitus Type 2, and hyperlipidemia. Various imaging modalities can be used to confirm the presence of steatosis.
4. Exclusion of other common chronic liver disorders with mild elevations in transaminases is a prerequisite to diagnosis. Alcohol abuse must be carefully evaluated by history and, if necessary, by carbohydrate-deficient transferrin screening and/or liver biopsy.
5. Treatment is simple, but difficult. It requires a change in lifestyle aimed at decreasing insulin resistance.

# Key References

1. Farrell GC, Larter CZ. Nonalcoholic fatty liver disease: from steatosis to cirrhosis. *Hepatology.* 2006;43(2 Suppl 1):S99-S112.
2. Vuppalanchi R, Chalasani N. Nonalcoholic fatty liver disease and nonalcoholic steatohepatitis: Selected practical issues in their evaluation and management. *Hepatology.* 2009;49(1):306-317.
3. Wieckowska A, Feldstein AE. Diagnosis of nonalcoholic fatty liver disease: invasive versus noninvasive. *Semin Liver Dis.* 2008;28(4):386-395.

# CHAPTER 36

# ALCOHOLIC LIVER DISEASE

Saro Khemichian, MD and
John A. Donovan, MD

Two-thirds of American adults drink some amount of alcohol. A subgroup tends to drink excessively, and this may lead to a number of alcohol-related conditions including alcoholic liver disease (ALD).

## Risk Factors

ALD does not necessarily follow a dose-dependent progression. Only a subset of heavy drinkers develop liver disease. Certain risk factors have been identified that promote the development and progression of ALD (Table 36-1). The amount of alcohol ingested is among the most important of these risk factors. The risk of developing alcoholic cirrhosis increases with ingestion of more than 60 to 80 g/day of alcohol in men and more than 20 g/day in women for 10 years or longer (Table 36-2).

## Diagnosis

The diagnosis of ALD begins with the identification of alcohol abuse. When social, psychological, or physiologic consequences of alcohol abuse are present, the identification of this disease is made more easily. However, clinicians often overlook important aspects of a pertinent history.

Esrailian E. *Gut Instincts: A Clinician's Handbook of Digestive and Liver Diseases* (pp 251-256).
© 2012 Taylor & Francis Group

| TABLE 36-1 | RISK FACTORS FOR THE DEVELOPMENT AND PROGRESSION OF ALCOHOLIC LIVER DISEASE |
|---|---|

- Male gender
- Race and ethnicity
- Presence of other liver diseases
- Type of alcohol consumed
- Binge drinking
- Genetic polymorphisms of genes involved in alcohol metabolism

| TABLE 36-2 | ALCOHOL VOLUME ASSOCIATED WITH ALCOHOLIC LIVER DISEASE | | |
|---|---|---|---|
| Type of Alcohol | Amount of Alcohol | Daily Intake Needed to Develop ALD in Men | Daily Intake Needed to Develop ALD in Women |
| Beer can (12 oz) | 9 to 13 g | 3 to 6 cans | 2 to 3 cans |
| Wine glass (4 oz) | 10 to 12 g | 4 to 8 glasses | 2 to 4 glasses |
| Hard liquor (1.5 oz) | 13 to 15 g | 3 to 6 drinks | 1 to 3 drinks |

There are many designed tools used to screen for alcohol abuse. The most commonly used of these is the CAGE questionnaire (Table 36-3). Two or more positive responses indicate problematic drinking. Although easy to administer, it has been criticized for focusing on the consequences of alcohol drinking rather than the amount of alcohol intake.

Physical examination findings may range from normal to the characteristic features of a more advanced chronic liver disease but are not always sensitive or specific to the diagnosis of ALD. One of the most common findings in ALD is hepatomegaly due to fatty infiltration of the liver. There are certain features of chronic liver disease that may be related to ALD. These include parotid gland enlargement, Dupuytren's contracture, and signs of feminization in men.

Liver enzyme and function testing may be normal in early ALD. Biomarkers exist to assess for more chronic alcohol abuse, but their application is limited. Measurement of the serum carbohydrate deficient transferrin (CDT) may be useful in the evaluation of the suspect patient who denies alcohol abuse. Bone marrow suppression caused by chronic alcohol use may manifest as neutropenia, anemia, or thrombocytopenia.

| TABLE 36-3 | CAGE QUESTIONNAIRE FOR ALCOHOL ABUSE |
|---|---|

1. Have you ever felt you should **C**ut down on your drinking?
2. Have people **A**nnoyed you by criticizing your drinking?
3. Have you ever felt bad or **G**uilty about your drinking?
4. Have you ever had a drink first thing in the morning (**E**ye opener) to steady your nerves or to get rid of a hangover?

Laboratory findings in more significant ALD include abnormalities in the liver panel. Aspartate aminotransferase (AST) results are usually less than 250 IU/L and more than 2 times the alanine aminotransferase (ALT) level. Other findings may indicate cirrhosis and portal hypertension. Hyperbilirubinemia, prolongation of the serum prothrombin time, and hypoalbuminemia reflect impaired hepatic excretory and synthetic functions. Thrombocytopenia, in the cirrhotic patient, is a usual result of hypersplenism.

Different imaging modalities such as ultrasound, computed tomography, and magnetic resonance imaging exist to assess for the presence of chronic liver disease, but none can diagnose ALD. Most imaging will show a liver enlarged by fatty infiltration in early disease and a cirrhotic liver with manifestations of portal hypertension in patients with more advanced disease.

Liver biopsy, not necessarily required to establish a diagnosis of ALD, can assist in determining the severity of liver injury or in the clarification of atypical cases. The typical histologies associated with spectrum of ALDs are detailed below. Alcoholic hepatitis features can also include ballooning degeneration of hepatocytes, alcoholic hyaline (Mallory bodies) within damaged hepatocytes, and infiltration by polymorphonuclear cells. Varying degrees of fibrosis may be seen with many patients demonstrating perisinusoidal fibrosis. Partial or complete obliteration of the terminal hepatic venule caused by centrilobular fibrosis is a characteristic pathology but not pathognomonic. Typical cirrhotic nodules in ALD tend to be micronodular or mixed micro- and macronodular.

# Spectrum of Alcoholic Liver Disease

## FATTY LIVER

Fatty liver is the earliest stage of injury to the liver as a result of alcohol. Steatosis is not specific to ALD, but fat accumulation in liver

| TABLE 36-4 | MODELS ASSESSING THE SEVERITY OF ALCOHOLIC HEPATITIS | |
|---|---|---|
| **Model** | **Equations/Variables Included** | **Utility** |
| Maddrey's Discriminant Function | 4.63 × prothrombin time (sec) + serum bilirubin (mg/dL) | Initiation of steroids/ prognosis |
| Model for End-Stage Liver Disease (MELD) | 9.57 × log creatinine (mg/dL) + 3.78 × log bilirubin (mg/dL) + 11.20 × log INR + 6.43 | Initiation of steroids/ prognosis |
| Glasgow Score | Age, WBC, PT, urea, bilirubin | Initiation of steroids/ prognosis |
| Lille model | Age, creatinine, bilirubin, PT, albumin, change in bilirubin level in 1 week | Stopping of steroids |
| INR indicates International normalized ratio; WBC, white blood cells; PT, prothrombin time | | |

cells can be a predictable response to alcohol ingestion. Alcoholic steatosis describes hepatocytes containing macrovesicular droplets of triglycerides and is the earliest type of injury seen in ALD. Patients at this stage are usually asymptomatic. Fatty liver caused by alcohol tends to be a benign condition that reverses with abstinence. The point that alcohol-related liver injury becomes irreversible is difficult to determine.

## ALCOHOLIC HEPATITIS

A subset of patients with ALD may present with acute alcoholic hepatitis. Most of these patients are chronic heavy drinkers, but many will have stopped drinking alcohol several weeks prior to presentation because of more acute illness. Typical findings include fever, jaundice, tender hepatomegaly, a bruit over the liver, and complications of portal hypertension. The patient with acute alcoholic hepatitis may also have other organ dysfunction such as pancreatitis and cardiomyopathy. Serum levels of AST are rarely above 300 IU/mL and are typically twice as high as ALT levels. Patients also have prolonged prothrombin time. Serum creatinine increase is often a sign of coexisting hepatorenal syndrome. Often, the diagnosis of alcoholic hepatitis is difficult because patients may have less typical presentations.

A variety of models have been developed to assess the severity of alcoholic hepatitis (Table 36-4). Most of these tools are associated with calculated scores that infer prognosis. These models are most important in assisting decisions related to the initiation or termination of treatments with identified benefits in the management of acute alcoholic hepatitis.

For the diagnosis of alcoholic hepatitis, several established treatments are available. The utility of each is determined by clinical situations. Corticosteroids are the most common medications used to halt the inflammatory process. Before embarking on corticosteroid treatment, it is of the utmost importance to rule out active infections. Prednisolone at a dose of 40 mg per day for 1 month is of proven benefit in the treatment of the uninfected patient with acute alcoholic hepatitis and Maddrey's Discriminant Function score (4.63 x prothrombin time [sec] + serum bilirubin [mg/dL]) of greater than 32. Calculation of the Lille score after 7 days of treatment indicates the utility of continuing corticosteroids. Response is most dependent on a significant decrease in the serum bilirubin. A Lille score greater than 0.56 indicates failed corticosteroid therapy and no benefit to continued treatment. Forty percent of patients are unresponsive to corticosterid treatment. There are no proven rescue therapies.

Pentoxifylline, presumably due to anti-tumor necrosis factor (TNF) properties, reduces short-term mortality among patients with alcoholic hepatitis. In a randomized prospective trial, this survival benefit was because of reduction in the incidence of the hepatorenal syndrome in the pentoxifylline-treated cohort. Most other studied anti-TNF agents have been ineffective in the treatment of alcoholic hepatitis. Supportive therapies include nutritional support and counseling for alcohol abstinence.

## ALCOHOLIC CIRRHOSIS

In some patients, chronic abuse leads to the progression of ALD to established cirrhosis and the complications of portal hypertension (varices, encephalopathy, ascites). Affected individuals are at an increased risk for liver disease-related death, hepatocellular carcinoma, or the need for liver transplantation. Continued alcohol drinking invariably leads to a worsened medical condition and an expected demise. Conversely, abstinence and a durable sobriety can result in clinical improvements and liver disease stability. The latter often affords the patient with decompensated cirrhosis the opportunity for liver transplantation if otherwise indicated. Most liver transplantation programs require at least 6 months of abstinence to qualify the patient with ALD for evaluation as a potential recipient.

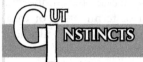

## ALCOHOLIC LIVER DISEASE

1. Alcohol abuse is a major cause of liver injury in the United States with a heavy burden on society.

2. Every clinician must screen for alcohol dependence and abuse. One of the most useful tools of screening is the CAGE questionnaire.

3. Liver histology can range from steatosis to sclerosing hyaline necrosis and cirrhosis.

4. Subset of patients with alcoholic hepatitis should be diagnosed and treated promptly based on clinical, laboratory, and prognostic models that have been developed.

5. Abstinence is the biggest key in treatment of ALD. Treatments for complications of chronic liver disease and special focus on nutrition of these patients go hand in hand.

# Key References

1. O'Shea RS, Dasarathy S, McCullough AJ; Practice Guideline Committee of the American Association for the Study of Liver Diseases, Practice Parameters Committee of the American College of Gastroenterology. Alcoholic liver disease. *Hepatology.* 2010;51(1):307-328.

2. Carithers RL, Mcclain CJ. Alcoholic liver disease. In: Feldman M, Feldman LS, Brandt LJ, eds. *Sleisenger and Fordtran's Gastrointestinal and Liver Disease: pathophysiology, diagnosis, management.* 9th ed. Philadelphia, PA: Saunders Elsevier; 2010:1383-1399.

3. Lucey MR, Mathurin P, Morgan TR. Alcoholic hepatitis. *New Engl J Med.* 2009;360(26):2758-2769.

4. Lefkowitch JH. Morphology of alcoholic liver disease. *Clin Liver Dis.* 2005;9(1):37-53.

# CHAPTER 37

# HEREDITARY LIVER DISEASES

Fasiha Kanwal, MD, MSHS

There are several liver disorders that result from inborn errors of metabolism. This chapter will cover hereditary metabolic diseases of the liver: hereditary hemochromatosis (HH), Wilson's disease, and α-1 antitrypsin deficiency (diagnostic tests summarized in Table 37-1) because these may be encountered by the practicing gastroenterologist.

## Hereditary Hemochromatosis

HH comprises several inherited disorders of iron homeostasis characterized by increased intestinal iron absorption that results in tissue iron deposition. The most common form of HH is hemochromatosis gene (HFE)-related HH. It is an autosomal recessive disorder and is the most common inherited disorder in the United States. Approximately 1 in every 200 to 300 White individuals in the United States are homozygous for the HFE gene mutation.

The HFE gene is located on the short arm of chromosome 6. The 2 common point mutations are C282Y and H63D. Approximately 90% of patients who present with HH are homozygous for C282Y, although some are compound heterozygotes (C282Y/H63D). However, clinically important iron overload can occur in the absence of HFE gene mutation.

Esrailian E. *Gut Instincts: A Clinician's Handbook of Digestive and Liver Diseases* (pp 257-264).

| TABLE 37-1 | TESTS USED IN THE DIAGNOSIS OF HEMOCHROMATOSIS, WILSON'S DISEASE, AND α-1 ANTITRYPSIN DEFICIENCY |
|---|---|
| **Condition** | **Tests** |
| Hereditary hemochromatosis | Serum iron and total iron binding capacity[1] |
| | Serum ferritin |
| | HFE gene mutation |
| | Liver biopsy[2] |
| Wilson's disease | Serum ceruloplasmin |
| | Slit-lamp examination for Kayser-Fleischer rings |
| | 24-hour urine copper |
| | Liver biopsy[3] |
| α-1 antitrypsin deficiency | α-1 antitrypsin phenotype |
| | Liver biopsy[3] |

[1]These tests are used to calculate the transferrin saturation (serum iron/total iron binding capacity x 100).
[2]A liver biopsy is not recommended for all patients with hemochromatosis. It is indicated in patients with serum ferritin >1000 ng/mL or with elevated liver enzymes in order to determine the stage of disease (such as presence of cirrhosis).
[3]In most cases, liver biopsy is necessary to confirm the diagnosis.

## CLINICAL PRESENTATION

Many patients with HFE-related HH are diagnosed as a result of abnormal serum iron studies during routine blood testing and are asymptomatic. Most patients with symptomatic HH are 40 to 50 years of age at the time of detection. Although C282Y homozygosity is equally distributed between men and women, clinical disease is less frequently encountered in women as a result of iron loss from normal menses and childbirth.

The typical symptoms include weakness, arthralgias, abdominal pain, and loss of libido or potency in men. Hepatomegaly is present in a majority of patients. Other manifestations relate to the level of iron overloading in nonhepatic organs and include diabetes mellitus, loss of libido and impotence, cardiomyopathy, arrhythmias, congestive heart failure, bronze discoloration of the skin, and arthropathy (HH-related arthropathy typically affects the second and third metacarpophalangeal joints). The bronze discoloration of skin in combination with diabetes led to the common term *bronze diabetes* that was used to describe HH.

## DIAGNOSIS

HH must be considered in any patient with typical symptoms or abnormal screening iron test results. If the history (including family history) and examination raise suspicion, then appropriate serum iron tests along with HFE gene mutation analysis should be obtained.

### Serum Iron Tests

Transferrin saturation (serum iron/total iron binding capacity x 100) of 45% or more is the earliest phenotypic presentation of HH. It is a more sensitive and specific test for HH than the second commonly employed iron test, serum ferritin. Serum ferritin can be normal in patients with HH and can be elevated in other inflammatory liver diseases. Therefore, ferritin alone should not be used as the initial screening test for HH.

### Hemochromatosis Gene Mutation Analysis

In patients with high transferrin saturation and serum ferritin, the next step in the diagnostic algorithm is to test for HFE gene mutation. Presence of a C282Y homozygous state confirms the diagnosis. Iron overload can also occur in a small proportion of patients with other HFE gene mutations, especially compound heterozygotes, which have a copy of C282Y and one copy of H63D, and occasionally in H63D homozygotes.

### Role of Liver Biopsy

With the advent of genetic testing, the need for liver biopsy in diagnosing HH has diminished. Liver biopsy is performed solely to assess the damage (if any) to the liver. If a patient is C282Y homozygote or a compound heterozygote (C282Y/H63D) and has serum ferritin less than 1000 ng/mL and normal liver enzymes, a liver biopsy is not needed. A liver biopsy is indicated in patients with serum ferritin more than 1000 ng/mL, patients with elevated liver enzymes, and in older patients with higher risk.

## TREATMENT AND PROGNOSIS

Most patients can be treated with routine phlebotomy and can tolerate weekly phlebotomy of 1 unit of whole blood. Weekly phlebotomies can continue until the hematocrit value drops below 37%. Transferrin saturation and ferritin levels can be checked at 2- to 3-month intervals to monitor response. When iron stores are depleted, as indicated by ferritin less than 50 ng/mL and transferrin saturation less than 50%, maintenance phlebotomies can be performed every 2 to 3 months with the goal to keep transferrin saturation below 50%. The iron chelating drug deferoxamine is used in patients who cannot tolerate phlebotomy. Patients will have a normal lifespan if treatment is initiated before development of significant fibrosis and cirrhosis. Established cirrhosis typically does not reverse with phlebotomy, and patients with cirrhosis continue to be at risk for hepatocellular cancer.

# Wilson's Disease

Wilson's disease is characterized by abnormal intrahepatic copper metabolism resulting in deposition of excess copper in the liver, brain, cornea, and other organs. It is an autosomal recessive disorder. Approximately 1/30,000 people are homozygous for a Wilson's disease mutation. The gene for Wilson's disease (ATP7B) is located on chromosome 13. Genetic testing is less useful for diagnosing Wilson's disease than for HH. In Wilson's disease, mutation of the ATP7B gene results in retention of copper in the liver and other organs.

## CLINICAL PRESENTATION

The clinical presentation of Wilson's disease is extremely variable. The age at the onset of presentation can range from 3 to 55 years. Patients may present with liver disease, a progressive neurological disorder without clinically prominent hepatic dysfunction, isolated acute hemolysis, or psychiatric illness.

Liver manifestations are more common in younger patients than in older patients and can present as chronic hepatitis, cirrhosis, or fulminant hepatic failure. Wilson's disease should be considered a possible diagnosis in all young patients with liver disease, although it is responsible for fewer than 5% of cases of chronic hepatitis in patients younger than 35 years old. Wilson's disease may present as fulminant hepatic failure (FHF). Acute intravascular hemolysis is usually present in patients with FHF, and renal failure may develop. Patients may present first with hemolytic anemia. Serum aminotransferases are lower than those seen in fulminant viral hepatitis, and serum alkaline phosphatase is usually normal or low. Total bilirubin level is disproportionately elevated due to hemolysis. Serum ceruloplasmin is not useful for making the diagnosis in patients with FHF. Urinary copper excretion is greatly elevated. These patients do not respond to medical therapy and require urgent liver transplantation. The combination of young age, severe liver dysfunction, and hemolytic anemia should be assumed to be Wilson's disease unless proven otherwise.

Neurological presentation tends to occur in the second and third decades and follows 2 main patterns—movement disorders and rigid dystonia. Psychiatric problems may range from depression and psychosis to subtle behavioral issues. Occasionally, the disease is identified incidentally due to ophthalmological findings. These include Kayser-Fleischer rings, which are brown rings at the periphery of the cornea due to copper deposition in the Descemet's membrane, and sunflower cataracts due to copper deposition in the lens. These are best identified during a slit-lamp examination. Kayser-Fleischer rings are present in only 44% to 62% of patients with mainly hepatic disease at the time of diagnosis but are almost invariably present in patients with a neurological presentation.

## DIAGNOSIS

Wilson's disease should be considered in any individual between the ages of 3 and 55 years with liver abnormalities of uncertain cause and must be excluded in any patient with unexplained liver disease along with neurological or neuropsychiatric disorders. The diagnosis is generally based on a slit-lamp examination for Kayser-Fleischer rings, testing for ceruloplasmin and urinary copper, and a liver biopsy.

### Slit-Lamp Examination

In a patient in whom Wilson's disease is suspected, Kayser-Fleischer rings should be sought by slit-lamp examination by a skilled examiner. The absence of Kayser-Fleischer rings does not exclude the diagnosis of Wilson's disease, even in patients with predominantly neurological disease.

### Serum Ceruloplasmin

A serum ceruloplasmin level of less than 200 mg/L (less than 20 mg/dL) has been considered consistent with Wilson's disease and is diagnostic if associated with Kayser-Fleischer rings. A level higher than 30 mg/dL essentially excludes the diagnosis of Wilson's disease except in patients with FHF.

### 24-Hour Urine Copper

Basal 24-hour urinary excretion of copper should be obtained in all patients in whom the diagnosis of Wilson's disease is being considered. The amount of copper excreted in the 24-hour period is typically more than 100 µg in symptomatic patients, but a finding of more than 40 µg may indicate Wilson's disease and requires further investigation.

### Liver Biopsy and Hepatic Copper Content

In most cases, liver biopsy is necessary to confirm the diagnosis. Hepatic copper content more than 250 µg/g dry weight remains the best biochemical evidence for Wilson's disease. A normal liver concentration of copper (less than 35 µg/g dry weight) excludes the diagnosis.

## TREATMENT AND PROGNOSIS

The recommended initial treatment of symptomatic patients is with chelating agents. The 2 chelating agents, D-penicillamine and trientine, work by eliminating excess copper. D-penicillamine is an effective first-line agent, but up to 20% of patients experience drug toxicity (hypersensitivity reactions, bone marrow suppression, proteinuria, autoimmune disorders, and dermatological conditions). Tolerability of D-penicillamine may be enhanced by starting with incremental doses, 250 to 500 mg/day, increased by 250-mg increments every 4 to 7 days to a maximum of 1000 to 1500 mg/day in 2 to 4 divided dosages. Maintenance dose is usually 750 to 1000 mg/day. Supplemental pyridoxine is provided at 25 to 50 mg by mouth daily to prevent vitamin $B_6$ deficiency.

Like penicillamine, trientine promotes copper excretion by the kidneys. Trientine is an effective treatment for Wilson's disease and is indicated especially in patients who are intolerant of penicillamine or have clinical features indicating potential intolerance. Trientine is given in doses similar to penicillamine and has few side effects. Occasionally, iron deficiency may develop because of sideroblastic anemia. Zinc acetate at 50 mg, 3 times daily, works by blocking copper uptake from the intestine. Zinc is currently reserved for maintenance treatment, pregnant patients, or those with pre-symptomatic disease.

Once disease symptoms or biochemical abnormalities have stabilized, typically in 2 to 6 months after initiation of therapy, maintenance dosages of chelators or zinc therapy can be used for treatment. Patients presenting without symptoms may be treated with either maintenance dosages of a chelating agent or with zinc from the outset.

# α-1 Antitrypsin Deficiency

α-1 antitrypsin deficiency is an autosomal co-dominant disease characterized by an increased risk of lung and liver disease. This deficiency is one of the most common genetic diseases in the world and the second most common metabolic disease affecting the liver. α-1 antitrypsin protects tissues from proteases such as neutrophil elastase and is encoded by a gene on the long arm of chromosome 14. Ninety-five percent of the population has the MM phenotype and is associated with normal serum levels of α-1 antitrypsin. The Z allele Pi*ZZ phenotype occurs in 1:2000 people, is associated with severe deficiency of α-1 antitrypsin, and is most clinically relevant for liver disease. The Pi*MZ phenotype leads to intermediate deficiency. In contrast to the lung disease that results from uninhibited effects of elastases and other proteolytic enzymes, liver disease results from accumulation of the mutant α-1 antitrypsin protein in the endoplasmic reticulum.

## CLINICAL PRESENTATION

α-1 antitrypsin deficiency may cause premature emphysema and liver disease. Most children with α-1 antitrypsin deficiency remain healthy during childhood. In adults, α-1 antitrypsin deficiency may cause hepatitis or chronic liver disease. Approximately 2% of adults with Pi*ZZ phenotype develop cirrhosis. Patients with cirrhosis due to α-1 antitrypsin deficiency are at a very high risk of hepatocellular cancer.

## DIAGNOSIS

The diagnosis of α-1 antitrypsin deficiency is made by α-1 antitrypsin phenotyping or genotyping. Unlike lung disease, liver disease does not correlate with the serum levels of α-1 antitrypsin. The diagnosis is confirmed by liver biopsy. The characteristic finding is the presence of eosinophilic, periodic acid-Schiff-positive, diastase-resistant globules in the endoplasmic reticulum of periportal hepatocytes.

## TREATMENT

There is no effective medical treatment for α-1 antitrypsin deficiency-associated liver disease. Patients should minimize alcohol use. Infusion of α-1 antitrypsin may be helpful for the lung disease, but it does not impact the liver disease. Liver transplantation is the only definitive liver treatment for α-1 antitrypsin deficiency. It cures the liver disease because the recipient assumes the Pi phenotype of the donor.

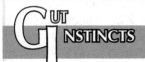

## HEREDITARY LIVER DISEASE

1. The diagnosis of HH must be considered in any patient with typical symptoms or abnormal screening iron test results. In patients with high transferrin saturation and serum ferritin, the next step is to test for HFE gene mutation. Presence of a C282Y homozygous state confirms the diagnosis.

2. Most patients with HH can be treated with weekly phlebotomy. When iron stores are depleted, as indicated by ferritin less than 50 ng/mL and transferrin saturation less than 50%, maintenance phlebotomies can be performed every 2 to 3 months, with the goal to keep transferrin saturation below 50%.

3. The clinical presentation of Wilson's disease is extremely variable. Patients may present with liver disease, a progressive neurological disorder without clinically prominent hepatic dysfunction, isolated acute hemolysis, or psychiatric illness.

4. A serum ceruloplasmin level less than 200 mg/L (less than 20 mg/dL) is diagnostic for Wilson's disease if associated with Kayser-Fleischer rings. In patients without Kayser-Fleischer rings, but with low serum ceruloplasmin and high urinary copper excretion, the diagnosis of Wilson's disease is confirmed by the presence of liver copper concentration greater than 250 µg /g dry weight.

5. The diagnosis of α-1 antitrypsin deficiency is made by α-1 antitrypsin phenotyping or genotyping. Liver transplantation is the only definitive treatment for α-1 antitrypsin deficiency.

## Key References

1. Bacon BR, Powell LW, Adams PC, Kresina TF, Hoofnagle JH. Molecular medicine and hemochromatosis: at the crossroads. *Gastroenterology.* 1999;116(1):193-207.

2. Roberts EA, Schilsky ML; American Association for Study of Liver Diseases (AASLD). Diagnosis and treatment of Wilson's disease: an update. *Hepatology.* 2008;47(6):2089-2111.

3. Eriksson S, Carlson J, Velez R. Risk of cirrhosis and primary liver cancer in alpha 1-antitrypsin deficiency. *N Engl J Med.* 1986;314(12):736-739.

# CHAPTER 38

# CHOLESTATIC LIVER DISEASES

Francisco Antonio Durazo, MD, FACP

## Primary Biliary Cirrhosis

### CLINICAL MANIFESTATIONS

Primary biliary cirrhosis (PBC) is characterized by chronic, nonsuppurative cholangitis affecting the interlobular and septal bile ducts. One unique feature is the high degree of specificity for involvement of the small intrahepatic ducts. The etiology of PBC is thought to be a combination of genetic predisposition and environmental triggers. Its clinical course can behave as a chronic cholestatic disease with a progressive course or may last many decades. The overall survival in patients treated with ursodeoxycholic acid (UDCA) without liver transplantation (OLT) is 84% at 10 years and 66% at 20 years. Serum bilirubin is the best predictor of survival. There is an increased risk of hepatocellular carcinoma (HCC) in patients with established cirrhosis.

Fatigue is the most common symptom and may be a manifestation of untreated hypothyroidism, which can be seen in 20% of patients with PBC. Pruritus can be seen in half of the patients and may diminish over time. It is worse at night and is often exacerbated by contact with wool, heat, or pregnancy. It can be incapacitating and is an indication for OLT. The cause is unknown, but seems to be due to increased opioidergic neurotransmission. Sicca syndrome is commonly seen in patients with PBC. Stigmata of itching, xanthelasma, and xanthomas are seen occasionally. Jaundice, vascular spiders, and signs of portal hypertension

Esrailian E. *Gut Instincts: A Clinician's Handbook of Digestive and Liver Diseases* (pp 265-272).
© 2012 Taylor & Francis Group

are seen in patients with advanced disease. Hyperpigmentation is common and possibly due to defective melanin degradation. Osteoporosis is seen in up to one-third of the patients. Hyperlipidemia with elevated high-density lipoprotein cholesterol is also common.

## DIAGNOSIS

The diagnosis of PBC should be entertained in any patient with cholestatic liver disease. Most patients will have elevations of alkaline phosphatase, mild elevations of the aminotransferases, increased levels of immunoglobulin M, serum bile acids, and serum cholesterol. Hyperbilirubinemia is an indication of more severe disease. Antimitochondrial antibodies (AMA) are present in 95% of the patients with PBC. Other autoimmune antibodies can also be present (antinuclear antibodies, smooth muscle antibodies).

Histology reveals nonsuppurative cholangitis affecting interlobular and septal bile ducts. Due to the high disease specificity of the mitochondrial antibodies, the role of liver biopsy in the diagnosis of PBC is questionable. Liver biopsy is recommended to confirm the diagnosis in AMA-negative PBC and to exclude other concomitant diseases, such as autoimmune hepatitis (AIH) or nonalcoholic steatohepatitis (NASH). The American Association for the Study of Liver Diseases (AASLD) Guidelines state that the diagnosis of PBC can be established when 2 of the following 3 criteria are met: (1) biochemical evidence of cholestasis based mainly on alkaline phosphatase elevation, (2) presence of AMA, and (3) histological evidence of nonsuppurative cholangitis and destruction of interlobular bile ducts. Patients with AMA-negative PBC are those who lack AMA, but whose clinical presentation, liver histology, and natural history are almost identical to patients with AMA-positive PBC. These patients have antinuclear and/or smooth muscle antibodies. Overlap of autoimmune hepatitis (AIH) with PBC can occur. The overlap features of PBC usually refer to simultaneous AIH in patients who have AMA-positive PBC. Patients with the overlap syndrome appear to have worse outcome because of complications related to the liver disease.

## TREATMENT AND FOLLOW UP

- PBC: UDCA 13 to 15 mg/kg/day in 2 divided doses for patients who have abnormal liver tests regardless of histological stage.
- Pruritus: Cholestyramine 4 g per dose to a maximum of 16 g/day given 2 to 4 hours before or after UDCA should be used as initial therapy. For pruritus refractory to cholestyramine: rifampin 150 mg to 300 mg twice daily, naltrexone 50 mg daily, or sertraline 75 to 100 mg daily.

- Sjogren's syndrome: Artificial tears, saliva substitutes, pilocarpine or cevimeline, and moisturizers for vaginal dryness.
- Surveillance for HCC with cross-sectional imaging and alphafetoprotein every 6 to 12 months.
- Bone disease: 1000 to 1500 mg of calcium and 1000 IU if vitamin D daily in the diet or as supplements if needed. Alendronate 70 mg weekly for osteopenic patients.
- Thyroid function testing.
- Upper endoscopy every 1 to 3 years to assess for esophageal varices.
- Liver transplantation for end-stage PBC.

# Primary Sclerosing Cholangitis

## CLINICAL MANIFESTATIONS

Primary sclerosing cholangitis (PSC) is a chronic, cholestatic liver disease characterized by inflammation and fibrosis of the intrahepatic and extrahepatic bile ducts, leading to the formation of multifocal bile duct strictures. It eventually develops into cirrhosis, portal hypertension, and hepatic decompensation in the majority of patients. Patients are at risk for the development of cholangiocarcinoma. PSC is more common in males and is strongly associated with inflammatory bowel disease (IBD) in 60% to 80% of patients. Conversely, PSC occurs in only 5% of patients with ulcerative colitis (UC) and in 3.4% of patients with Crohn's disease. Clinical symptoms include right upper quadrant discomfort, fatigue, pruritus, and weight loss.

## DIAGNOSIS

The diagnosis of PSC is made in patients with a cholestatic biochemical profile and a cholangiogram (magnetic resonance cholangiogram [MRC]), endoscopic retrograde cholangiogram (ERC), or percutaneous transhepatic cholangiogram (PTC) showing the characteristic bile duct changes with multifocal strictures and segmental dilatation. The clinical history, distribution of cholangiographic findings, and the presence or absence of IBD have to be taken into consideration when determining if an abnormal cholangiogram is due to PSC or a secondary process. Small-duct PSC is a variant characterized by typical cholestatic and histologic features of PSC, but normal bile ducts on cholangiogram. Patients with small-duct PSC have a better prognosis, less risk for cholangiocarcinoma (CCA), and 15% may evolve into classic PSC.

Cholangitis is an uncommon feature at presentation. Laboratory tests usually indicate cholestasis; however, a normal alkaline phosphatase does not exclude the diagnosis. A wide variety of autoantibodies can be detected in the serum of patients with PSC. They have no role in the routine diagnosis of PSC, including the perinuclear antineutrophil cytoplasmic antibody (p-ANCA), which is nonspecific. The ERC was regarded as the gold standard in diagnosing PSC. However, ERC is an invasive procedure with potentially serious complications. Magnetic resonance cholangiogram has become the diagnostic imaging modality of choice when PSC is suspected with a sensitivity and specificity of 80% or more and 87% or more, respectively, for the diagnosis of PSC. However, it should be noted that patients with early changes of PSC may be missed by MRC, and ERC still has a useful role in excluding large-duct PSC where MRC views may not be optimal. Liver biopsy may show periductal concentric (onion skin) fibrosis, the classic histopathologic finding of PSC, but this observation is infrequent and may also be seen in secondary sclerosing cholangitis. A liver biopsy is not required to make the diagnosis of large-duct PSC if the cholangiogram is abnormal. It is essential in the diagnosis of suspected small-duct PSC and for the assessment of possible overlap syndromes (PSC-AIH). The PSC-AIH overlap syndrome is characterized by clinical, biochemical, and histological features of AIH in the presence of cholangiographic findings identical to PSC.

## RISK OF MALIGNANCY

Patients who have IBD and PSC are at increased risk of colorectal cancer (CRC) and dysplasia compared with patients with UC alone. CRC associated with PSC appears to have a predilection for the right colon. Surveillance colonoscopy at 1- or 2-year intervals from the time of diagnosis of PSC in patients with UC is recommended. Due to the increased risk of CRC in Crohn's colitis, patients with PSC who have Crohn's disease (CD) are recommended to be surveyed similarly to patients with UC.

Patients with PSC are prone to develop gallbladder cancer. There is a high risk of malignancy associated with gallbladder polyps. An annual ultrasound to detect mass lesions in the gallbladder is recommended. In patients with gallbladder mass lesions, a cholecystectomy is recommended, regardless of lesion size, if the underlying liver disease permits. Patients with PSC are also at risk for developing CCA. The risk factors include hyperbilirubinemia, variceal bleeding, proctocolectomy, UC with CRC or dysplasia, the duration of IBD, and polymorphisms of the NKG2D gene. Contrary to the risk of neoplasia in IBD, the duration of PSC does not seem to be a risk factor for the development of CCA. In half the patients with PSC and CCA, the malignancy is detected at the time of diagnosis or within the first year. The diagnosis of superimposed CCA in PSC is challenging because of the presence of strictures and inflammation inherent to the disease. Cancer antigen (CA) 19-9 with a cut-off of 130 U/mL has been used for surveillance of CCA in PSC patients with a sensitivity and specificity of 79% and 98%, respectively. However, CA 19-9 can be elevated in patients with bacterial cholangitis and is virtually undetectable in 7% of the normal population.

The demonstration of a mass lesion with characteristic imaging features has virtually a 100% sensitivity and specificity for the diagnosis of CCA. However, visible mass lesions on imaging are unusual in early stage CCA. Ultrasonography, computed tomography, and magnetic resonance imaging, in the diagnosis of CCA in PSC patients, yielded an overall positive predictive value of 48%, 38%, and 40%, respectively. Endoscopic retrograde cholangiopancreatography and magnetic resonance cholangiopancreatography have an overall positive predictive value for CCA of only 23% and 21%, respectively. Direct visualization with cholangioscopy and intraductal ultrasound are promising technologies for the diagnosis of CCA, but have not yet been tested in large patient populations nor validated by multiple studies. Conventional brush cytology by ERCP has a sensitivity that ranges from 18% to 40% and a specificity of 100%. There are no guidelines for the surveillance of CCA in PSC patients due to the lack of evidence-based information. Many clinicians screen PSC patients with an imaging study plus a CA 19-9 annually.

## TREATMENT

### Endoscopic Therapy

The goal of the endoscopic or percutaneous approach in patients with PSC is to relieve biliary obstruction. Patients with dominant strictures (stenosis with a diameter of 1.5 mm or less in the common bile duct or 1 mm or less in the common hepatic duct), cholangitis, jaundice, right upper quadrant pain, or worsening liver tests are appropriate candidates for therapy. Stricture dilatation can be performed with balloon or coaxial dilators. It can be performed periodically with or without stenting. However, biliary stenting has been shown to be associated with increased complications when compared to endoscopic dilatation only, and it should be reserved for strictures that are refractory to dilatation. Prophylactic antibiotics should be used routinely during ERC in PSC patients. In regard to surgical treatment, no data have shown that either bypass or resection of a dominant stricture affect natural history of disease progression.

### Medical Therapy

UDCA has shown biochemical improvement but no effect on disease progression and complications of portal hypertension. High-dose UDCA (28 to 30 mg/kg/day) was associated with serious adverse events, particularly in advanced disease. Thus, the role for UDCA in slowing the progression of PSC-related liver disease is as yet unclear. Treatment with corticosteroids and other immunosuppressant agents has not demonstrated any improvement in disease activity or in outcome.

### Metabolic Bone Disease

Hepatic osteodystrophy is common in patients with PSC. Patients with PSC should have a bone density examination to exclude osteopenia or osteoporosis at diagnosis and at 2- to 3-year intervals. Patients with hepatic osteopenia should be treated with calcium 1.0 to 1.5 g and vitamin D 1000 IU daily. Patients with osteoporosis should be given biphosphonate therapy, in addition to calcium and vitamin D. In patients with esophageal varices, it is recommended to use parenteral forms of biphosphonate therapy rather than oral formulations.

### Liver Transplantation

Indications for liver transplantations in patients with PSC do not differ substantially from other forms of chronic liver disease and relate primarily to the complications of portal hypertension. The 5-year survival is 85%, and the impact of recurrent PSC in the graft remains controversial.

### Cholangiocarcinoma

Patients with PSC and CCA in the absence of cirrhosis should be considered for surgical resection. If the patient is not a good candidate for resection because of significant underlying liver disease, or because the tumor is unresectable, he or she should be considered for liver transplantation with neoadjuvant radiochemotherapy by experienced transplant centers.

## Secondary Sclerosing Cholangitis

Sclerosing cholangitis refers to a spectrum of chronic, progressive diseases of the intra- and/or extrahepatic bile ducts characterized by patchy inflammation, fibrosis, and stricturing. Clinical and cholangiographic findings identical to PSC have been described in patients with different inflammatory, infectious, and oncologic diseases (Table 38-1). It is important to be aware of these conditions and have in mind that not all sclerosing cholangitis is primary.

| TABLE 38-1 | MOST COMMON DISEASE ASSOCIATIONS WITH SCLEROSING CHOLANGITIS |
|---|---|
| Inflammatory bowel disease | Ulcerative colitis<br>Crohn's disease |
| Idiopathic fibrosis | Retroperitoneal fibrosis<br>Mediastinal fibrosis<br>Peyronie's disease<br>Idiopathic lobular panniculitis |
| Autoimmune and connective tissue disorders | Systemic lupus erythematosus<br>Celiac disease<br>Rheumatoid arthritis<br>Sjögren's syndrome<br>Type 1 diabetes mellitus<br>Immunoglobulin G4-related cholangitis |
| Infections | Cholangitis |
| Secondary etiology | Cholelithiasis<br>Choledocolithiasis |
| Immunodeficiency-related | Acquired immunodeficiency syndrome |
| Pancreatic diseases | Autoimmune pancreatitis<br>Chronic pancreatitis |
| Toxic | Intraductal formaldehyde<br>Hypertonic saline<br>Intra-arterial chemotherapy |
| Ischemic | Hepatic allograft arterial occlusion<br>Post-traumatic sclerosing cholangitis |

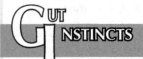

## CHOLESTATIC LIVER DISEASE

1. Antimitochondrial antibodies are present in 95% of the patients with PBC.

2. A liver biopsy is not required to make the diagnosis of large-duct PSC if the cholangiogram is abnormal.

3. UDCA 13 to 15 mg/kg/day should be used in 2 divided doses for PBC irrespective of normal liver tests.

4. Surveillance colonoscopy at 1- or 2-year intervals from the time of diagnosis of PSC in patients with UC or Crohn's colitis is recommended.

5. Patients with PSC and cholangiocarcinoma in the absence of cirrhosis should be considered for surgical resection.

## Key References

1. Kaplan M, Gershwin M. Primary biliary cirrhosis. *N Engl J Med.* 2005; 353(12):1261-1273.

2. Chapman R, Fevery J, Kalloo A, et al. Diagnosis and management of primary sclerosing cholangitis. *Hepatology.* 2010;51(2):660-678.

3. Abdalian R, Heathcoate E. Sclerosing cholangitis: a focus on secondary causes. *Hepatology.* 2006;44(5):1063-1074.

# CHAPTER 39

# Autoimmune Hepatitis

Vivian Ng, MD and
Sammy Saab, MD, MPH, AGAF

Autoimmune hepatitis (AIH) is a chronic inflammatory disease of the liver of unknown etiology and is characterized by the presence of specific histological changes, circulating auto-antibodies, and hyper-gammaglobulinemia. AIH can occur in patients of all ages, and women are affected more than men.

## Pathogenesis

The pathogenesis involves a cascade of events that occurs in genetically predisposed individuals. An environmental agent is believed to trigger the process that leads to AIH. The exact relationships between genes and the autoimmune process remain largely undefined, but certain viruses and drugs have been identified as potential triggering agents. The specific autoantigens remain unidentified but are under investigation.

## Clinical Manifestations

Clinical manifestations can range from completely asymptomatic patients to those with fulminant hepatic failure. A period of subclinical disease may occur prior to presentation. Patients can present with varied symptoms including pruritis, fatigue, lethargy, malaise, abdominal pain, nausea, or arthralgias. Several extrahepatic disorders have been associated with AIH. They include ulcerative colitis, hemolytic anemia,

Esrailian E. *Gut Instincts: A Clinician's Handbook of Digestive and Liver Diseases* (pp 273-280).
© 2012 Taylor & Francis Group

idiopathic thrombocytopenic purpura, diabetes mellitus, thyroiditis, Grave's disease, celiac disease, systemic lupus erythematosus, rheumatoid arthritis, and skin diseases such as vitiligo and Sweet's syndrome.

# Classification of Autoimmune Hepatitis

### TYPE 1

Type 1 AIH, also known as classic AIH, is most commonly associated with circulating antibodies to nuclei (ANA) and/or smooth muscle. Antibodies to soluble liver antigens (SLA) occur in approximately 10% to 30% of patients. This is the most common form of AIH in the world and affects all age groups.

### TYPE 2

Type 2 AIH, more common in Europe and some South American countries, is characterized by antibodies to liver/kidney microsomes (ALKM-1) and/or to a liver cytosol antigen (ALC-1). Type 2 AIH is much more common in the pediatric population.

### TYPE 3

Type 3 AIH is the least described form. These patients do not have the typical auto-antibodies seen in Type 1 or Type 2 AIH. The antibody that defines Type 3 AIH is the soluble liver antigen/liver pancreas (anti-SLA/LP). Type 3 AIH typically affects females, typically occurs between the ages of 20 and 40, and may rapidly progress to cirrhosis.

### VARIANTS OF AUTOIMMUNE HEPATITIS

Overlaps between AIH with primary biliary cirrhosis (PBC) and primary sclerosing cholangitis (PSC) have been widely recognized as variants of AIH. Patients with variant forms have serologic findings consistent with AIH in addition to findings of other forms of chronic liver disease, such as PBC or PSC. There are 2 subtypes of the PBC-AIH variants: (1) serologic findings of PBC, with detectable antimitochondrial antibodies (AMA), and (2) histologic findings suggestive of PBC, but seronegative for AMA. Patients with AIH and overlap with PSC have serologic findings of AIH along with cholangiographic abnormalities consistent with PSC.

| TABLE 39-1 | ANTIBODIES IN AUTOIMMUNE HEPATITIS | |
|---|---|---|
| **First Line** | **Second Line** | **Third Line** |
| Antinuclear antibodies (ANAs) | Liver/kidney microsome Type 1 (LKM-1) | Protoplasmic-staining anti-neutrophil cytoplasmic antibodies (pANCA) |
| Smooth muscle antibodies (SMAs) | Soluble liver antigen/liver pancreas (SLA/LP) | Asialoglycoprotein receptor (ASGPR) |
| | | Liver-specific cytosol antigen Type 1 (LC1) |

# Diagnosis

Diagnosis is based on the presence of characteristic serologic and histologic findings and also the exclusion of other forms of liver disease. Histologically, AIH is characterized by a portal plasma cell infiltrate that invades the hepatocyte boundary surrounding the portal triad and infiltrates into the surrounding lobule, also known as interface hepatitis. Bile duct changes, including destruction, cholangitis, or ductopenia, are present in a portion of the cases. Fibrosis is also typically seen except in the mildest form of AIH. Cirrhosis can be found with progressive AIH.

Typically, the degree in elevation of aminotransferase values is greater than the elevation of bilirubin and alkaline phosphatase. Increased levels of gamma globulins and immunoglobulin G (IgG) are commonly seen in AIH. Auto-antibodies must be present, and the conventional ones include ANA, smooth muscle antibody (SMA), and anti-liver/kidney microsome Type 1 (LKM1). Other antibodies can help support a probable diagnosis if other conventional markers are negative (Table 39-1).

# Serologic Markers

ANA is the traditional marker and is present alone or with SMA in 67% of patients with AIH. Anti-smooth muscle antibody (SMA) is found less often than ANA. Anti-LKM1 typically occurs in the absence of ANA and SMA. Protoplasmic-staining antineutrophil cytoplasmic antibody (pANCA) is common in AIH, but does not have diagnostic specificity nor prognostic implications in AIH. Newer antibodies are currently being evaluated. Other antibodies such as antibodies to asialo-glycoprotein receptor (anti-ASGPR), liver-specific cytosol antigen Type 1 (anti-LC1), soluble liver antigen/liver pancreas (anti-SLA/LP), actin, or pANCA can help support a diagnosis of AIH if other conventional markers are negative.

# Treatment

Treatment should be based on severity of symptoms, degree of elevation in serum aminotransferase levels, and histologic findings on liver biopsy. The elevation in aminotransferase and IgG levels does not necessarily correlate with the extent of histologic injury.

The American Association for the Study of Liver Diseases (AASLD) recommends instituting treatment for patients with serum aminotransferases greater than 10-fold the upper limit of normal or for patients with aminotransferases that are 5-fold greater than the upper limit of normal along with a serum gamma globulin level greater than twice the upper limit of normal. In addition, patients with histologic findings of bridging necrosis or multiacinar necrosis warrant therapy. In patients not meeting the above criteria, treatment should be individualized and based on clinical judgment. Histologic findings of interface hepatitis without bridging necrosis or multiacinar necrosis should not prompt treatment. In addition, treatment may not be indicated in patients with inactive cirrhosis, pre-existing comorbid conditions, or drug intolerances. Lastly, in most children, treatment is warranted at time of diagnosis.

Corticosteroids, the mainstay of treatment in AIH, have demonstrated a survival benefit in patients with severe disease on histology. Steroid-sparing therapy with azathioprine or 6-MP is also frequently used (Figure 39-1). Combination regimens allow the use of lower doses of corticosteroids and may reduce the corticosteroid-related side effects. Azathioprine or 6-MP is typically avoided in patients with pre-existing cytopenias, malignancy, and thiopurine methyltransferase deficiency. Other steroid-sparing medications include mycophenolate mofetil, cyclosporine, and tacrolimus (Table 39-2). The combination of prednisone and azathioprine (or 6-MP) is the preferred initial treatment because of the lower frequency of side effects from prednisone alone. However, these agents can be associated with bone marrow suppression. Patients not treated should be monitored closely, including repeating liver biopsies, for disease progression every 2 years.

Remission is defined as the resolution of symptoms, reduction in serum aminotransferase levels to less than twice the upper limit of normal, improvement of serum bilirubin and gamma globulin levels, and repeat liver histology showing improvement to normal or mild portal hepatitis. Practically, the goal is to have liver enzyme normalization. Although most patients will have biochemical improvement within weeks of therapy, histologic improvement may take up to 3 to 6 months. Therefore, remission is typically not seen before 12 months, and a fixed dose of daily maintenance medication should be used until remission

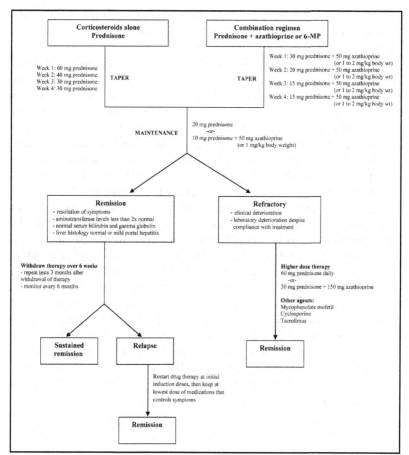

**Figure 39-1.** AIH treatment algorithm.

| TABLE 39-2 | MEDICATIONS USED IN AUTOIMMUNE HEPATITIS |
|---|---|
| **First Line** | **Second Line** |
| Prednisone | Mycophenolate mofetil |
| Azathioprine | Tacrolimus |
| 6-Mercaptopurine | Cyclosporine |

is achieved. After achieving remission, corticosteroids should be withdrawn gradually, and patients should be monitored with serial clinical visits and laboratory tests.

Treatment failure is seen in approximately 10% of patients with deterioration despite compliance. It is noted that treatment failure is more frequent in patients with established cirrhosis, those with disease at a younger age or longer duration of disease before therapy is initiated, or patients who possess the human histocompatibility (HLA)-B8 and/or the HLA-DR3 phenotypes. Treatment with higher doses of therapy can help achieve remission within 2 years. Other immunosuppressant therapy, such as cyclosporine, tacrolimus, and mycophenolate mofetil, should be considered in patients refractory to azathioprine/6-MP.

Relapse is common after cessation of drug therapy, and up to 50% of patients require repeat therapy for recurrent disease. Relapse typically occurs within the first 15 to 20 months after withdrawal of therapy. Following the first relapse, drug therapy should be reinitiated at induction doses, and drug withdrawal should be attempted once again after remission is achieved. In patients with more than 2 episodes of relapse, long-term maintenance therapy is recommended with the lowest dose of prednisone or azathioprine. A small number of patients who are refractory to treatment develop end-stage liver disease and require liver transplantation. Five-year patient and graft survival after liver transplantation ranges between 83% and 92%, whereas 10-year survival is approximately 75%. Patients are still at risk for recurrent AIH after liver transplantation and require close monitoring.

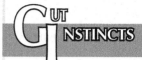

## AUTOIMMUNE HEPATITIS

1. AIH is a chronic inflammation of the liver, characterized by circulating auto-antibodies, hypergammaglobulinemia, and histologic changes, and can occur in children and adults of all ages.

2. Serologic abnormalities include elevated aminotransferase levels, elevated serum gamma globulin levels, and auto-antibodies such as ANAs, SMAs, and anti-LKM1s. Newer auto-antibodies such as anti-ASGPR, anti-LC1, anti-SLA/LP, anti-actin, or pANCA can help support a probable diagnosis if other conventional markers are negative.

3. Characteristic histologic changes in AIH consist of periportal hepatitis with lymphocytic infiltrates, plasma cells, and piecemeal necrosis, which can progress to bridging necrosis and panlobular necrosis.

4. Treatment includes corticosteroids, or corticosteroids in conjunction with steroid-sparing therapy such as azathioprine or 6-MP. Combination doses of corticosteroids and azathioprine/6-MP may reduce the corticosteroid-related side effects.

5. Remission is the resolution of symptoms, normalization of serologies, and improvement on repeat liver histology. Serologic improvement can be seen within 2 weeks of therapy; however, histologic improvement may take up to 3 to 6 months. A fixed dose of daily maintenance medication should be used until remission is achieved.

# Key References

1. Czaja AJ, Freese DK, American Association for the Study of Liver Disease. Diagnosis and treatment of autoimmune hepatitis. *Hepatology*. 2002;36(2): 479-497.

2. Krawitt EL. Autoimmune hepatitis. *N Engl J Med*. 2006;354(1):54-66.

3. Manns MP, Vogel A. Autoimmune hepatitis, from mechanisms to therapy. *Hepatology*. 2006;43(2 Suppl 1):S132-S144.

CHAPTER 40

# Complications of Portal Hypertension

Bruce A. Runyon, MD

Most patients in the United States with portal hypertension have cirrhosis. Although cirrhosis is the 12$^{th}$ leading cause of death in the United States in general, it is the fourth leading cause of death of people between the ages of 45 and 54. Most patients who die due to cirrhosis die from one or more of the complications of cirrhosis, detailed here. The "big 3" complications are ascites, hepatic encephalopathy (HE), and variceal hemorrhage. Development of hepatorenal syndrome is part of the natural history of ascites in many patients. Treatment of the liver disease that is the cause of these complications can dramatically improve or resolve the complication(s). In particular, alcoholic cirrhosis with or without alcoholic hepatitis can improve dramatically with abstinence even if hepatitis C or another insult to the liver is present. Table 40-1 describes general strategies to improve survival in patients with cirrhosis. Baclofen (5 mg orally, 3 times daily for 3 days; then 10 mg, 3 times daily) has been shown in a randomized trial to reduce alcohol craving and consumption. This author has had great success with baclofen for this indication and essentially no side effects in this population. Decompensated hepatitis B cirrhosis can respond dramatically to (non-interferon-based) antiviral therapy. Other causes of cirrhosis are less reversible.



Esrailian E. *Gut Instincts: A Clinician's Handbook of Digestive and Liver Diseases* (pp 281-288).
© 2012 Taylor & Francis Group

| TABLE 40-1 | GENERAL STRATEGIES TO IMPROVE SURVIVAL IN PATIENTS WITH CIRRHOSIS |
|---|---|

- Abstinence from alcohol
- Treat the cause(s) of cirrhosis when possible
- Minimize medications
- Avoid nephrotoxic and hepatotoxic medications
- Avoid aspirin and other nonsteroidal anti-inflammatory drugs (NSAIDs)
- Acetaminophen and tramadol are the main pain relievers in cirrhosis
- Hydroxyzine and trazodone are safe sedatives in patients with cirrhosis
- Avoid narcotics and benzodiazepines
- Advise patients against eating raw oysters and clams
- Avoid surgical procedures and perform minimally invasive procedures instead, or avoid invasion altogether
- Avoid prophylactic diets. Sodium should not be restricted until there is fluid retention. Protein is almost never restricted
- Perform screening endoscopy for esophageal varices and prescribe nonselective beta blocker prophylaxis if large varices are detected
- Perform an ultrasound and a computed tomography scan of the abdomen yearly and an alfa-fetoprotein test twice yearly

# Ascites

Ascites is the most common complication of cirrhosis, developing in 47% of patients within 10 years of detection of compensated cirrhosis (ie, cirrhosis without evidence of a complication). Approximately 85% of patients with ascites have cirrhosis. A diagnostic abdominal paracentesis with cell count, differential, and serum-ascites albumin gradient is required to rule in portal hypertension (serum-ascites albumin gradient 1.1 g/dL or more) and rule out infection. If the absolute neutrophil count is 250/cu mm or more, empiric treatment with a third-generation cephalosporin (such as cefotaxime 2 g intravenously every 8 hours for 5 days) is indicated. If an organism is isolated that is susceptible to a narrower-spectrum antibiotic, treatment can be altered accordingly.

The remaining 15% of causes for ascites include peritoneal carcinomatosis, heart failure, alcoholic hepatitis, and miscellaneous.

## TREATMENT

First-line treatment of ascites in the setting of cirrhosis includes 2 g/day sodium diet, diet education of the patient and the cook, and dual diuretics, usually starting with single morning doses of 100 mg daily of spironolactone and 40 mg of furosemide. Dosing more than once per day invites noncompliance and reduces efficacy. Spironolactone is actually more efficacious than furosemide in cirrhosis. Both drugs are usually needed. Random urine sodium/potassium ratios help assess response to treatment. Patients with a urine sodium greater than urine potassium should be losing weight. If they are not losing weight, attention should be given to better dietary compliance. Treatment options for those who excrete an inadequate amount of urine sodium, and hence, do not lose weight despite maximum tolerated doses of diuretics, include liver transplantation, serial large-volume-paracentesis, and transjugular intrahepatic portosystemic shunt (TIPS). Also, there is some evidence that midodrine can revert diuretic-resistant ascites back to diuretic sensitive by increasing renal perfusion pressure. The dose can be started at 5 mg orally, 3 times daily, and titrated upward to increase blood pressure and natriuresis. Hypertension is rare in truly diuretic-resistant patients.

# Hepatorenal Syndrome

In the absence of a reversible or treatable component, cirrhosis usually slowly and silently progresses. Patients regularly transition from a compensated state to diuretic-responsive ascites to diuretic-resistant ascites and then on to hepatorenal syndrome (HRS). HRS can develop slowly in this fashion (Type 2), or it can be rapidly precipitated by an insult that perturbs the hyperdynamic circulation of these patients (Type 1), such as spontaneous bacterial infection or variceal hemorrhage. Patients can develop Type 1 HRS in the setting of Type 2 HRS. Until the late 1990s, HRS was considered the final complication of cirrhosis with survival measured in days to weeks. Now, with vasoconstrictor treatment plus albumin infusion and successful treatment of the precipitating cause, Type 1 HRS can reverse, and renal function can return to the level prior to the Type 1 HRS episode. Most patients (70% to 80%) diagnosed with HRS actually do not have it. Instead, they have diuretic-induced azotemia, drug-induced renal injury, underlying chronic renal disease, or a combination of these lesions. The key to an accurate diagnosis is a careful search for recent exposure to potentially offending drugs, fluid weight loss, blood loss, serial measurements of the basic metabolic panel, urinalysis, and renal ultrasound.

TREATMENT

Type 1 HRS may respond to albumin infusion and octreotide/midodrine administration. Other drugs are under evaluation.

# Hepatic Encephalopathy

HE is the second most common complication of cirrhosis, developing in 28% of patients within 10 years of detection of compensated cirrhosis. This is characterized by reversible confusion that can initially be very subtle but can progress to coma. It is regularly precipitated by narcotics, sedatives, benzodiazepines, gut hemorrhage, bacterial infection, or volume depletion. Patients with cirrhosis regularly complain of insomnia. Hydroxyzine 25 mg at night is the only data-supported sedative in cirrhosis. Trazodone 100 mg can also be tried. More typical sedatives are poorly tolerated by patients prone to HE.

The most refractory cases occur after TIPS or portocaval shunt surgery.

TREATMENT

Protein restriction should not be used as treatment of HE. Protein restriction further aggravates the malnutrition, which is already predictably present and may actually worsen the confusion. First-line treatment consists of enough oral lactulose to produce 2 to 3 stools daily. If the patient is too comatose to drink safely, lactulose can be given by enema.

Rifaximin may be used to supplement or replace lactulose. It is available in a 550-mg pill and is administered twice daily. Patients who are refractory to first-line treatment (with or without rifaximin) can be given neomycin 1 g orally twice daily. The amount of time spent confused or comatose can lead to dementia. Some patients who have had severe HE prior to liver transplantation may have persistent mental status changes after transplant.

# Variceal Hemorrhage

Variceal hemorrhage (VH) is the third most common complication of cirrhosis, developing in 25% of patients within 10 years of detection of compensated cirrhosis. This condition can be prevented by performing a surveillance endoscopy and placing all patients with large varices on prophylactic nonselective beta blockers. Variceal hemorrhage is characterized by hematemesis and/or melena. Up to 50% of patients with cirrhosis and upper gut bleeding bleed from a source other than esophageal varices. The esophagus is the usual site where varices bleed when they are the source of bleeding. Approximately one-third of patients who develop upper gut bleeding in the setting of cirrhosis have taken aspirin or a similar drug within 2 weeks. Patients with cirrhosis should be instructed to completely avoid such drugs except for the rare patient in whom the cardiac or cerebral perfusion status is more serious than the cirrhosis.

Acetaminophen is well tolerated as a minor pain reliever in cirrhosis with a maximum dose of 4000 mg daily. Patients with cirrhosis may be relatively protected from the hepatotoxicity of acetaminophen; the active agent is a metabolite, which patients with cirrhosis may be slow to produce.

## TREATMENT

Patients with cirrhosis and evidence of upper gut bleeding should be brought to the hospital by ambulance, resuscitated, transfused to a target hemoglobin of 7 to 8 g/dL, given octreotide at 50 mcg per hour infusion, and rapidly endoscoped. If esophageal varices have bleeding stigmata and no other source is evident, band ligation should be performed. This author has found that placing as many bands as possible on esophageal varices with each session minimizes bleeding between sessions as well as the number of sessions. If varices are so small that only 4 to 6 bands are placed in the first session, those varices were probably not the source of hemorrhage. Repeat banding should be performed every other week until variceal obliteration. This usually takes a total of three sessions. Proton pump inhibitors (PPIs) are given twice daily until 30 days after the last banding; then, they are discontinued. Long-term PPIs can increase risk of bacterial infections including *Clostridium difficile* in patients with cirrhosis.

# Hepatocellular Carcinoma

Hepatocellular carcinoma (HCC) is the terminal complication of cirrhosis that patients develop if they live long enough and do not die of something else. Lifetime risk approaches 20%. Chronic hepatitis C, hepatitis B, nonalcoholic steatohepatitis-related cirrhosis, and iron overload appear to be the highest risk for HCC. Alcohol-related cirrhosis appears to be of intermediate risk. Primary biliary cirrhosis and cirrhosis due to autoimmune hepatitis or Wilson's disease appear to be lowest risk for HCC.

As patients are kept alive longer with state-of-the-art treatment and even prevention of complications of cirrhosis, this malignant tumor is being detected with increasing frequency. The "epidemics" of chronic hepatitis C and obesity are also contributing to the increasing numbers of patients with HCC. Hepatitis B and nonalcoholic steatohepatitis can be complicated by HCC even before cirrhosis develops. Even children (younger than 10 years old) with hepatitis B can develop HCC with genotype F.

Patients with cirrhosis should receive imaging (eg, ultrasound and a computed tomography scan yearly) and measurement of alpha-fetoprotein (AFP) in serum every 6 months to detect HCCs at early treatable stages.

## TREATMENT

Too often, screening is not performed until symptoms of an advanced HCC are present, and treatment options are very limited at that point. These patients may die even before they can receive the only data-supported systemic chemotherapy that prolongs life with HCC—sorafenib. This is an oral form of chemotherapy that is quite expensive and requires frequent (even weekly, initially) clinic visits to prevent and treat the peculiar and potentially disabling rash and diarrhea that may develop.

Some focal lesions are detected in the 5- to 20-mm size range with regular surveillance. Repeating imaging and AFP testing every 3 months can help determine which of these small lesions is malignant and which is simply a macroregenerative nodule. Magnetic resonance imaging may also be useful in the differential diagnosis. However, screening with magnetic resonance imaging may visualize many nodules that prove to be benign after an extensive evaluation. This modality is better reserved for differential diagnosis of a focal lesion found on another type of image.

Treatment options for tumors larger than 20 mm in maximum dimension include radiofrequency ablation, chemoembolization, proton radiation (in centers that have large accelerators), as well as heating and cryoablation techniques. Local expertise usually determines which option a given patient receives. Surgical resection in the setting of cirrhosis is seldom tolerated. Because the entire liver is premalignant, resecting a portion does not solve the basic problem and exposes the patient to postoperative morbidity and mortality. Patients who survive resection too often develop new HCCs. In the United States, chemoembolization is the most common treatment modality. Patients who are liver transplant candidates should be evaluated for that treatment option. If there is no extrahepatic tumor at the time of transplant, this option can be curative.

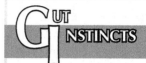

**PORTAL HYPERTENSION**

1. First-line treatment of ascites in the setting of cirrhosis includes sodium-restricted diet, spironolactone, and furosemide. Second-line treatment includes liver transplantation, serial large-volume paracentesis, and transjugular intrahepatic portasystemic shunt.
2. HE can be avoided by minimizing narcotic, benzodiazepine, and sedative use.
3. HE is treated by lactulose or rifaximin. Neomycin can be added for refractory cases.
4. Variceal hemorrhage can be prevented by endoscopically screening for varices and prescribing nonselective beta blockers for large varices. Variceal hemorrhage is treated by transfusion, vasoconstrictors, and urgent banding.
5. HCC is detected early by screening imaging and testing alpha-fetoprotein levels.

## Key References

1. Runyon BA. Diagnosis and evaluation of patients with ascites. In: Basow DS, ed. *UpToDate*. Waltham, MA: UpToDate, Inc; 2010.
2. Runyon BA. Management of adult patients with ascites due to cirrhosis: an update. *Hepatology*. 2009;49(6):2087-2107.
3. Gines P, Qunitero E, Arroyo V, et al. Compensated cirrhosis: natural history and prognostic factors. *Hepatology*. 1987;7(1):122-128.

# ABNORMAL LIVER TESTS
# IN PREGNANCY

Vandana Khungar, MD, MSc and
Tram T. Tran, MD

Abnormal liver tests in pregnancy lead to frequent hepatology consultations. Expedient and correct interpretation of these tests can both reassure the patient and clinician and, if needed, lead to early intervention to prevent complications. Table 41-1 summarizes the interpretation of liver tests in various clinical scenarios in pregnancy.

## Hyperemesis Gravidarum

### DIAGNOSIS

Hyperemesis gravidarum (HG) is intractable vomiting in the first trimester of pregnancy, typically between 4 and 10 weeks of gestation that necessitates the use of intravenous hydration. Risk factors include hyperthyroidism, psychiatric illness, molar pregnancy, pre-existing diabetes, and multiple pregnancies. Fifty percent of patients experience aminotransferase elevation up to 20 times the upper limit of normal, and jaundice is occasionally present. Viral hepatitis must be ruled out in this setting as HG is a clinical diagnosis. Liver biopsy is rarely needed. If performed, the histology is normal or shows bland cholestasis.

Esrailian E. *Gut Instincts: A Clinician's Handbook
of Digestive and Liver Diseases* (pp 289-296).
© 2012 Taylor & Francis Group

## TABLE 41-1

## INTERPRETATION OF LIVER TESTS IN PREGNANCY

| Disease or Health State | AST | ALT | Bile Acids | Bilirubin | Alkaline Phosphatase | Uric Acid | Platelets | PT/PTT | Urine Protein |
|---|---|---|---|---|---|---|---|---|---|
| Not pregnant | 7 to 40 IU/L | 0 to 40 | 5 to 10 | 0 to 17 | 30 to 130 | Normal | Normal | Normal | Normal |
| 1st trimester | 10 to 28 | 6 to 32 | 5.1 to 5.4 | 4 to 16 | 32 to 100 | Normal | Normal | Normal | Normal |
| 2nd trimester | 10 to 29 | 6 to 32 | 5.3 to 5.7 | 3 to 13 | 43 to 135 | Normal | Normal | Normal | Normal |
| 3rd trimester | 11 to 30 | 6 to 32 | 5.6 to 6.5 | 3 to 14 | 133 to 418 | Normal | Normal | Normal | Normal |
| Hyperemesis gravidarum | 1 to 2x ULN | 1 to 2x ULN | Normal | <5 mg/dL | 1 to 2x | Normal | Normal | Normal | Normal |
| ICP | 1 to 4x | 1 to 4x | 30 to 100x | <5 mg/dL | 1 to 2x | Normal | Normal | Normal | Normal |
| AFLP | 1 to 5x | 1 to 5x | Normal | <10 mg/dL | 1 to 2x | Increased | Sometimes decreased | Sometimes increased | Sometimes increased |
| Pre-eclampsia/ eclampsia | 1 to 100x | 1 to 100x | Normal | <5 mg/dL | 1 to 2x | Increased | Sometimes decreased | Sometimes increased | Increased |
| HELLP | 1 to 100x | 1 to 100x | Normal | <5 mg/dL | 1 to 2x | Increased | Decreased | Sometimes increased | Sometimes increased |
| Hepatic rupture | 2 to 100x | 2 to 100x | Normal | Sometimes increased | Increased | Normal | Sometimes decreased | Sometimes increased | Normal |

AST indicates aspartate aminotransferase; ALT, alanine aminotransferase; PT/PTT, prothrombin time/partial thromboplastin time; ICP, Intrahepatic cholestasis of pregnancy; AFLP, acute fatty liver of pregnancy; HELLP, hemolysis, elevated liver enzymes, low platelets; ULN, upper limit of normal.

## TREATMENT

Treatment of HG includes hospitalization for rehydration, nutritional support, and symptom control with antiemetics and occasionally steroids.

# Intrahepatic Cholestasis of Pregnancy

## PATHOPHYSIOLOGY

Intrahepatic cholestasis of pregnancy (ICP) results from abnormal biliary transport across the canalicular membrane resulting in pruritus and elevated bile acid levels with onset in the second half of pregnancy and normalization of laboratory values after delivery. It is the second most common cause of jaundice in pregnant women, with viral hepatitis being the most common. There may be a genetic predisposition to ICP, and a mutation in the MDR3 (ABCB4) gene is associated with the disorder. ICP recurs in only 45% to 70% of pregnancies. Fetal complications include placental insufficiency, premature labor, and sudden fetal death likely due to elevated fetal levels of bile acids. Fetal bile acids are transported across the placental membrane to the maternal circulation; high maternal levels of bile acids are associated with fetal morbidity and mortality.

## DIAGNOSIS

Pruritus usually starts at approximately 25 to 32 weeks of gestation, affects all parts of the body, and is occasionally worse at night. Aminotransferase levels vary from mildly elevated to 10- to 20-fold elevations, bilirubin is usually less than 5 mg/dL, alkaline phosphatase is elevated, but is not helpful in diagnosis in pregnancy. Elevated levels of gamma-glutamyl transferase are found in less than 30% of cases. The most specific and sensitive marker of ICP is serum bile acid levels of greater than 10 micromol/L and can be elevated 100-fold. Diagnosis in the first pregnancy is presumptive, made on clinical suspicion alone, and can be confirmed with rapid postpartum resolution. Elevated serum bile acid levels help to make the diagnosis but are not available at all hospitals. Liver biopsy is used only to rule out more serious conditions.

## TREATMENT

ICP is managed with symptomatic therapy for the mother, close monitoring of the fetus, and early delivery when possible. Pruritus and liver dysfunction resolve immediately after delivery with no maternal mortality. Prior to delivery, withdrawal of exogenous progesterone can cause remission of pruritus. Fat-soluble vitamin supplementation can be given at the time of delivery in those with severe steatorrhea. The treatment of choice is ursodeoxycholic acid (UDCA) in doses of 10 to 15 mg/kg body weight, as it provides relief of pruritus in some patients, improvement in liver tests, improved fetal outcome with less prematurity, and no adverse maternal or fetal effects. Dexamethasone (1 mg/day for 7 days) is less effective than UDCA but does promote fetal lung maturity. S-adenosyl-L-methionine is also less effective but may have an additive effect. ICP resolves with delivery, but recurs in 45% to 70% of subsequent pregnancies and sometimes with oral contraceptives.

# Pre-eclampsia and HELLP Syndrome

Pre-eclampsia consists of hypertension, edema, and proteinuria in the third trimester and occurs in 5% to 10% of all pregnancies. Involvement of the liver indicates severe pre-eclampsia and is the most common cause of hepatic tenderness and aminotransferase elevations in pregnancy. Aminotransferases vary from mild to 10- to 20-fold elevations, and bilirubin is usually less than 5 mg/dL. Hemolysis (H), elevated liver tests (EL), and low platelet counts (LP) constitute the HELLP syndrome. In 2% to 12% of cases of severe pre-eclampsia, HELLP syndrome may also occur in conjunction with the pre-eclampsia.

## PATHOPHYSIOLOGY

HELLP syndrome is a microangiopathic hemolytic anemia leading to areas of hemorrhage and necrosis from zone 1 to involve the whole lobule, with hematomas, capsular tears, and intraperitoneal bleeding. Most patients present between 27 and 36 weeks gestation, but up to 25% present in the postpartum period.

## DIAGNOSIS

Diagnosis of HELLP requires the presence of all 3 lab criteria: hemolysis, elevated aminotransferases, and thrombocytopenia. Maternal complications are common, including diffuse intravascular coagulation (DIC), abruptio placentae, acute renal failure, eclampsia, pulmonary edema, acute respiratory distress syndrome, severe ascites, subcapsular hematoma, hepatic failure, and wound hematomas.

## TREATMENT

Delivery of the infant is the treatment of choice and will usually result in resolution of the pre-eclampsia and HELLP syndromes, but liver transplantation has been performed in those with persisting bleeding from a hematoma, hepatic rupture, or liver failure from extensive necrosis. Perinatal mortality is 11%.

# Acute Fatty Liver of Pregnancy

## PATHOPHYSIOLOGY

Acute fatty liver of pregnancy (AFLP) occurs in the third trimester of pregnancy with microvesicular fatty infiltration resulting in hepatic encephalopathy and failure. It sometimes involves abnormalities in intramitochrondrial fatty acid oxidation. Beta-oxidation of fatty acids in hepatic mitochondria requires long-chain 3-hydroxyacyl-CoA dehydrogenase (LCHAD), and mutations in this gene are closely associated with AFLP; LCHAD deficiency has been identified in 20% of babies of mothers with AFLP.

## DIAGNOSIS

In patients with AFLP, 40% to 50% of are nulliparous and there is an increased incidence in twin pregnancies. AFLP occurs in the third trimester from 28 to 40 weeks and rarely in the late second trimester or postpartum period. The usual clinical presentation involves 1 to 2 weeks of anorexia, nausea, vomiting, headache, and right upper quadrant pain, jaundice, hypertension, edema, ascites, a small liver, and hepatic encephalopathy. Fifty percent of patients with AFLP have pre-eclampsia, and there is some overlap with the HELLP syndrome. In AFLP, aminotransferases vary from near-normal to 1000, usually about 300 to 500; bilirubin is usually less than 5 mg/dL, but higher in severe disease. Other laboratory abnormalities include anemia, leukocytosis, normal to low platelets, coagulopathy with or without DIC, metabolic acidosis, renal dysfunction, hypoglycemia, high ammonia, and pancreatitis. A presumptive clinical diagnosis and biopsies are usually not performed due to coagulopathy and the need for urgent therapy. Definitive diagnosis is histological with microvesicular fatty infiltration from free fatty acids predominantly in zone 3 with lobular disarray and mild portal inflammation with cholestasis. The differential diagnosis of acute liver failure in the third trimester is AFLP, HELLP, and fulminant viral hepatitis. Patients with AFLP are more likely to have liver failure with coagulopathy, hypoglycemia, encephalopathy, DIC, and renal failure than those with HELLP syndrome.

## TREATMENT

AFLP must be treated with immediate delivery and intensive support-ive care for the mother and baby. There has never been a report of recov-ery prior to delivery. Caesarean section is usually performed, but vaginal delivery will reduce the incidence of major intra-abdominal bleeding. Two to 3 days after delivery, the aminotransferases and encephalopathy improve, but intensive supportive care is needed. Most patients improve 1 to 4 weeks postpartum, but a cholestatic phase with rising bilirubin and alkaline phosphatase can persist for longer. Recovery is usually complete with no signs of chronic liver disease. Maternal mortality is 7% to 18%, and fetal mortality is 9% to 23%. Liver transplantation is considered only in those who advance to fulminant hepatic failure after the first 1 to 2 days postpartum without signs of hepatic regeneration. Women who are LCHAD carriers have an increased risk of recurrence in 20% to 70% of all pregnancies.

# Coincidental Liver Disease in a Pregnant Patient

## VIRAL HEPATITIS

Hepatitis due to A, B, C, D, E, herpes simplex, cytomegalovirus, and Epstein-Barr viruses accounts for 40% of jaundice in pregnant women in the United States. Hepatitis A, B, and C occur in the same frequency in the pregnant and nonpregnant populations and during each trimester of pregnancy. Hepatitis E is very rare in the United States, but endemic to Asia, Africa, and Central America. It can become fulminant in the third trimester with up to 25% mortality. Herpes simplex hepatitis presents as a severe or fulminant "anicteric" hepatitis in the third trimester and can be treated with acyclovir or vidarabine. Supportive care is instituted for acute viral hepatitis. It is not an indication for termination of pregnancy, caesarean section, or to not breastfeed.

All pregnant women should be screened for hepatitis B as part of their first trimester screening tests. If they are at high-risk and not immune, they can receive the vaccine while pregnant. Perinatal trans-mission of hepatitis B is highest in those with acute hepatitis, particu-larly HBeAg-positive patients. Transmission of hepatitis B rarely occurs transplacentally, but more likely at the time of delivery. Transmission is preventable in 95% of cases by passive-active immunoprophylaxis of babies at birth with hepatitis B immunoglobulin (HBIG) and hepatitis B virus vaccine. Vertical transmission of hepatitis A and D can occur with high viral loads at the time of delivery. Transmission of hepatitis C to the baby is 1% to 5%, with numbers in the higher range if the mother has HIV co-infection, abuses intravenous drugs, and has maternal viremia greater than $10^6$ copies/mL. Transmission of hepatitis C is not affected by mode of delivery or breastfeeding. If a mother has hepatitis A during the third trimester, the baby should be given passive immuno-prophylaxis with immune globulin within 48 hours of birth.

## GALLSTONES AND BILIARY DISEASE

Cholesterol secretion increases in the second and third trimesters compared to bile acids and phospholipids, leading to supersaturated bile, cholesterol crystals, biliary sludge, and gallstones. Up to 10% of pregnant patients develop gallstones, but only 0.1% to 0.3% of women experience symptoms in the form of biliary colic, gallstone pancreatitis, and acute cholecystitis. Laparoscopic cholecystectomy during the second trimester is indicated in patients with intractable biliary colic, severe acute cholecystitis not responding to supportive treatment, or acute gallstone pancreatitis.

## CHRONIC LIVER DISEASE IN THE PREGNANT PATIENT

In hepatitis C, aminotransferases can fall, and viral ribonucleic acid can increase during pregnancy with the reverse occurring in the postpartum period. Immunosuppression should be continued during pregnancy for autoimmune hepatitis. Flares can be treated with increased steroids and azathioprine. Patients with Wilson's disease should continue to be treated to avoid fulminant disease. Patients with advanced cirrhosis and portal hypertension are usually amenorrheic and infertile due to hypothalamic-pituitary dysfunction, but pregnancy can occur in those with compensated cirrhosis and mild portal hypertension. Increased fetal loss and variceal bleeding (in 20% to 25%) of cirrhotic patients occurs. Other risks include hepatic decompensation, jaundice, thrombocytopenia, and rupture of splenic aneurysms. Patients who have had a liver transplant can plan for pregnancy beyond the first 2 years after transplant and still have excellent outcomes. There is, however, risk of fetal prematurity, acute rejection, or recurrent viral hepatitis.

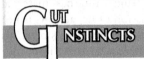

## LIVER TESTS IN PREGNANCY

1. The most common cause of jaundice in pregnancy in the United States is viral hepatitis.

2. ICP is the second most common cause of jaundice in pregnant women.

3. Pregnancy-specific liver diseases occur as follows: first trimester, HG; second trimester, ICP and pre-eclampsia/eclampsia; third trimester, ICP, pre-eclampsia/eclampsia, AFLP, and HELLP syndrome.

4. Abnormal liver tests occur in 3% to 5% of pregnancies, most of which is pregnancy related, but can occur in an asymptomatic patient or in nonhepatic diseases in pregnancy.

5. Cirrhosis reduces fertility, but if a cirrhotic patient becomes pregnant, the mother is at risk for complications of portal hypertension and should be managed by a hepatologist.

## Key References

1. Hepburn IS. Pregnancy-associated liver disorders. *Dig Dis Sci.* 2008;53(9): 2334-2358.

2. Hay JE. Liver disease in pregnancy. *Hepatology.* 2008;47(3):1067-1076.

3. Lee NM, Brady CW. Liver disease in pregnancy. *World J Gastroenterol.* 2009;15(8):897-906.

# FULMINANT LIVER FAILURE AND TRANSPLANTATION

John P. Duffy, MD

Fulminant hepatic failure (FHF) is a clinical syndrome consisting of jaundice, encephalopathy, and coagulopathy in patients without history of liver dysfunction. It is an aggressive disease process requiring intensive care therapeutics and, often, urgent liver transplantation (LT) as a life-saving measure. The overall mortality rate for patients presenting with FHF nears 50%, and FHF now accounts for about 5% of all LTs performed. Clinicians must be familiar with FHF to implement rapid therapy and to initiate early transfer to a LT center for supportive care, transplant evaluation, and liver replacement.

## Definitions

Several forms of acute liver failure have been described. FHF has been defined as the development of encephalopathy within 2 weeks of the onset of jaundice. Acute liver failure (ALF) classically refers to the development of jaundice, encephalopathy, and coagulopathy within 8 weeks of onset of illness. Subfulminant hepatic failure refers to acute liver failure complicated by encephalopathy within 2 to 12 weeks of jaundice. All of these forms of liver failure are characterized by the absence of prior liver disease. Acute hepatic decompensation describes acute worsening of liver function in patients with previously compensated chronic liver disease (usually secondary to infection, bleeding, electrolyte imbalance, or other stressors). The aim of this chapter is to discuss the recognition, evaluation, and treatment of patients with FHF.

Esrailian E. *Gut Instincts: A Clinician's Handbook
of Digestive and Liver Diseases* (pp 297-302).
© 2012 Taylor & Francis Group

# Etiology

FHF can result from a variety of insults to the liver, including drug toxicity (acetaminophen), viral hepatitis (hepatitis A/B), metabolic disorders (Wilson's disease), vascular problems (Budd-Chiari syndrome), idiosyncratic drug reactions (amoxicillin/clavulanic acid), other toxins (*Amanita* mushrooms, aflatoxin), and complications of pregnancy. In most series in the United States, acetaminophen overdose and viral hepatitis are the most common causes of FHF, accounting for 30% and 15% of cases, respectively. In one of the largest single-center series of patients transplanted for FHF, more than 50% of patients had cryptogenic FHF, whereas 17% had viral hepatitis, 13% had acetaminophen toxicity, and 11% had drug-induced FHF. Cryptogenic FHF is more common among children, and, in fact, in the largest collection of children transplanted for FHF, 70% of cases were cryptogenic, 12% were related to acetaminophen overdose, and 12% were related to hepatitis A infection.

# Diagnosis

FHF can present as acute onset of mental status changes and rapidly progressive multi-organ dysfunction, or it can evolve in a slower, more insidious manner, but still ultimately resulting in liver failure and death. Patients without prior liver disease who present with new transaminitis, jaundice, coagulopathy, metabolic acidosis, and renal dysfunction should be strongly suspected of having FHF and should be admitted, monitored, treated with aggressive supportive care, and referred to a transplant center. Encephalopathy usually is a late finding and can herald a trajectory of accelerated clinical deterioration. It cannot be emphasized strongly enough that any patient with a suspected diagnosis of FHF should be referred immediately to an LT center for further care, urgent evaluation, and listing. LT is often the only effective treatment for FHF, and any delay can significantly worsen a patient's prognosis. The clinical course of FHF can be highly unpredictable, and it is not unusual for coherent, alert patients to become comatose, hypoglycemic, and in multisystem organ failure in only a matter of hours. LT should be thought of as a safety net for patients with FHF; it can always be avoided if a patient demonstrates signs of clinical recovery, but it cannot be used as a life-saving endeavor unless the patient has been fully evaluated and is actively listed for LT at an experienced center.

Several prognostic models have been developed to predict which patients will require LT for FHF. The best known are the King's College Criteria, which are predictors of poor outcome in patients with FHF (Table 42-1). In the King's College experience, etiology of FHF

| TABLE 42-1 | KING'S COLLEGE CRITERIA—PREDICTORS OF POOR OUTCOME FROM FULMINANT HEPATIC FAILURE |
|---|---|
| Acetaminophen-induced FHF | pH <7.30 (irrespective of grade of encephalopathy) OR<br><br>All of the following:<br>• PT >100 sec (INR >6.5)<br>• Serum creatinine >3.4 g/dL<br>• Stage III or IV hepatic encephalopathy |
| Non-acetaminophen-induced FHF | PT >100 sec (INR >6.5) (irrespective of grade of encephalopathy) OR<br><br>Any 3 of the following (irrespective of grade of encephalopathy):<br>• Age less than 10 or greater than 40 years<br>• Etiology: non-A, non-B hepatitis, halothane hepatitis, drug toxicity<br>• Duration of jaundice to encephalopathy >7 d<br>• PT 50 sec (INR 3.5)<br>• Serum bilirubin >17.5 g/dL |

was the most important prognostic factor; patients with acetaminophen overdose had better chance of medical recovery than did patients with FHF from other causes. Patients who satisfy the King's College criteria are considered to have a 95% chance of mortality with only supportive therapy. Therefore, these patients require LT as life-saving treatment. However, most transplant physicians can recount numerous patients initially outside the criteria progressing to life-threatening FHF or, conversely, deathly-ill patients meeting the criteria, but spontaneously recovering.

## Medical Treatment

While awaiting transfer to an LT center, supportive care is critical. Most patients require intravenous fluids for volume resuscitation and correction of acidosis. Severe coagulopathy (international normalized ratio [INR] >3) should be addressed with infusion of fresh-frozen plasma and administration of vitamin K. For patients with acetaminophen toxicity, immediate therapy with either intravenous or enteral acetylcysteine (initial bolus of 140 mg/kg, followed by 70 mg/kg every

4 hours x 16 doses) should be initiated. Some liver centers use the acetylcysteine protocol for all patients with FHF, regardless of etiology, and some continue dosing the medication beyond 16 doses. Recent experience with the intravenous form of acetylcysteine has been quite encouraging and is well tolerated by patients.

Major complications of FHF include infection and sepsis, so patients diagnosed with FHF should be started on broad-spectrum antibiotics. Renal function should be closely monitored, and severe metabolic acidosis refractory to volume resuscitation should be treated with early renal replacement therapy. Correction of coagulopathy may be required for attainment of vascular access and, therefore, the decision on renal replacement therapy needs to be made as early as possible.

Cerebral edema and herniation are common causes of death for patients with rapid deterioration from FHF. Patients with FHF should receive an early noncontrast computed tomography (CT) of the brain, and this study should be repeated for any signs of worsening neurologic status. Intravenous support should be directed with isotonic to hypertonic fluids to avoid hyponatremia, which can exacerbate cerebral edema. Significant neurologic deterioration (confusion, lethargy, stupor, severe agitation) should be addressed with early endotracheal intubation and sedation as needed. Once this has occurred, intracranial pressure (ICP) monitoring and serial brain CT scans are necessary to follow the neurologic status. As with dialysis access, correction of coagulopathy is critical prior to insertion of ICP monitors, and safe implantation usually requires an INR less than 1.5 and platelets greater than 50,000. Medical measures should be employed to keep the ICP less than 15 mm Hg and the cerebral perfusion pressure greater than 50 mm Hg, and elevation of the head and hyperventilation should be used to keep the $pCO_2$ level between 25 and 30 mm Hg. Diuresis with mannitol and furosemide can be used provided the serum osmolality is less than 320 mOsm/L. Sedation with propofol can be helpful, and some patients require pentobarbital coma for progressive cerebral edema. Patients with significant cerebral edema are often placed on seizure prophylaxis with levetiracetam (Keppra) as the antiepileptic of choice, but the American Association for the Study of Liver Diseases guidelines do not currently have a formal recommendation for prophylactic antiepileptic therapy.

## Liver Transplantation

For patients with irreversible FHF, LT is the only definitive therapy. Deciding whether or not to transplant a patient with FHF offers great challenges, especially in patients with a chance to recover. An aggressive approach toward listing and activating patients with FHF is favored, and then declining transplantation if real signs of recovery develop. Frequent monitoring of liver function (serial INR, neurologic assessments) is crucial during this period to stratify patients with regard to transplantation versus medical therapy. Moreover, patients with FHF can often present complex ethical challenges, especially in patients with suicidal overdoses, polysubstance abuse, or other psychosocial issues. An inclusive, multidisciplinary approach to LT is favored, unless the patient has shown a consistent pattern of behavior and/or abuse that is incompatible with full recovery and post-transplant compliance.

The urgent nature of the transplant can mandate the use of extended criteria organs as a life-saving attempt. Hepatitis B core antibody positive grafts and even ABO mismatch grafts can be used to replace the liver in a patient who would otherwise die with FHF. Living donor LT is generally applicable only in an adult-to-pediatric arrangement. Most adults with toxic FHF do not achieve metabolic correction with a split liver graft.

Overall 1- and 5-year survival rates after LT for FHF are 75% and 68% (patient) and 64% and 57% (graft), respectively. For pediatric recipients, 1- and 5-year survival rates are 81% and 77% (patient) and 77% and 73% (graft), respectively. While multiple series have identified prognostic factors for LT in patients with FHF, pretransplant renal function appears to be the single most important predictor of post-transplant outcome, with poor renal function associated with poorer patient and graft outcomes. In patients transplanted for FHF, sepsis and multi-organ failure are the main causes of post-transplant death, and primary nonfunction is the most common cause of early graft loss.

## Summary

LT is the only definitive treatment for FHF, and 5-year post-transplant survival is approximately 70%. As a result, early transfer to an LT center is mandatory once FHF is diagnosed.

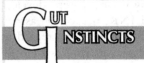

## FULMINANT LIVER FAILURE

1. Patients with irreversible FHF who will require LT as a life-saving therapy almost always manifest the clinical syndromes of coagulopathy, acidosis, and renal failure.
2. Improving trends in serum transaminase levels do not imply improvement in liver function.
3. Some patients may recover from the initial hepatic insult, but chronically manifest progressive cholestasis after resolution of the transaminitis. Patients should be followed closely by liver transplant teams until the serum bilirubin and international normalized ratio begin to normalize.
4. The development of seizures in the setting of FHF portends a poor prognosis, even after LT.
5. Patients with suspected FHF, even in the absence of encephalopathy, should be transferred as early as possible to institutions specializing in LT.

## Key References

1. O'Grady JG, Alexander GJ, Hayllar KM, Williams R. Early indicators of prognosis in fulminant hepatic failure. *Gastroenterology.* 1989;97(2):439-445.
2. Farmer DG, Anselmo DM, Ghobrial RM, et al. Liver transplantation for fulminant hepatic failure: experience with more than 200 cases over a 17-year period. *Ann Surg.* 2003;237(5):666-676.
3. Farmer DG, Venick RS, McDiarmid SV, et al. Fulminant hepatic failure in children: superior and durable outcomes in children over 25 years at a single center. *Ann Surg.* 2009;250(3):484-493.

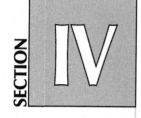

SECTION IV

# ENDOSCOPY

# CHAPTER 43

# SEDATION

Jeremy M. Wong, MD and
Samuel H. Wald, MD

While many endoscopic procedures were once performed without sedation, more than 98% in the United States are now routinely performed under sedation. Properly administered sedation will not only optimize conditions for the endoscopist, but it can improve safety and patient satisfaction. Sedation-related complications with endoscopy can account for up to half of the serious adverse events.

The American Society of Anesthesiologists (ASA) has published practice guidelines that describe 4 levels of sedation, ranging from mild sedation (anxiolysis) to general anesthesia (Table 43-1). Due to significant variability in patient response and the narrow therapeutic window of some medications, practitioners must be prepared for and trained in the resuscitation of a patient who reaches a deeper level of sedation than originally planned. Most endoscopic procedures are performed under moderate sedation (also referred to as conscious sedation). In this level of sedation, a patient should have a purposeful response to verbal or tactile stimulation (note that reflex withdrawal from a painful stimulus is not a purposeful response). If a patient has become purposely responsive only after repeated or painful stimulation, he or she has progressed into deep sedation, and practitioners must be able to recognize and treat the complications that may arise until the patient has regressed back to a lighter plane of sedation, such as maneuvers of airway rescue to open the airway and supportive ventilation as necessary.

Esrailian E. *Gut Instincts: A Clinician's Handbook
of Digestive and Liver Diseases* (pp 305-312).
© 2012 Taylor & Francis Group

| TABLE 43-1 | CONTINUUM OF DEPTH AND SEDATION: DEFINITION OF GENERAL ANESTHESIA AND LEVELS OF SEDATION/ANALGESIA | | | |
|---|---|---|---|---|
| | Minimal Sedation (Anxiolysis) | Moderate Sedation/ Analgesia (Conscious Sedation) | Deep Sedation/ Analgesia | General Anesthesia |
| Responsiveness | Normal response to verbal stimulation | Purposeful* response to verbal or tactile stiulation | Purposeful* response after repeated or painful stimulation | Unarousable even with painful stimulus |
| Airway | Unaffected | No intervention required | Intervention may be required | Intervention often required |
| Spontaneous ventilation | Unaffected | Adequate | May be inadequate | Frequently inadequate |
| Cardiovascular function | Unaffected | Usually maintained | Usually maintained | May be impaired |

*Reflex withdrawal from a painful stimulus is not considered a purposeful response. (Reprinted with permission from American Society of Anesthesiologists Task Force on Sedation and Analgesia by Non-Anesthesiologists. Practice guidelines for sedation and analgesia by non-anesthesiologists. *Anesthesiology.* 2002;96:1004-1017.)

Deep sedation should only be administered by providers comfortable with delivering general anesthesia safely. Such a provider should be trained in supporting a patient's airway, ventilation, and cardiovascular function. In some patients, it may be advised to have intravenous sedation under monitored anesthesia care (MAC) or general anesthesia provided by an anesthesiologist.

## Preparation for Sedation

All patients should have a documented preprocedure history and physical so the anesthetic plan may be optimized to decrease the risk of adverse outcomes for both moderate and deep sedation. The history should include questions about previous adverse experience with sedation/anesthesia. A focused physical examination should include a complete airway evaluation. In women of childbearing age, the possibility of pregnancy should be discussed.

Using the ASA Classification system, many patients who are ASA I to III may safely undergo sedation without the need for an anesthesiologist. ASA IV to V patients, patients undergoing emergency procedures, patients with evidence of airway difficulties (congenital malformation, history of head/neck irradiation or surgery, sleep apnea, advanced rheumatoid arthritis/cervical spine disease, morbid obesity, small mouth opening), history of alcohol or substance abuse, pregnancy, severe neurologic or neuromuscular disease, history of problems with conscious sedation in the past, or patients undergoing more complex procedures (endoscopic ultrasound, endoscopic retrograde cholangiopancreatography, stent placement in the upper gastrointestinal tract, upper gastrointestinal endoscopy with drainage of pseudocyst) should be considered for MAC or general anesthesia by an anesthesiologist.

While there is no consensus regarding preprocedural fasting due to a lack of data, the ASA guidelines recommend for healthy patients undergoing elective procedures a 2-hour fast after clear liquids (water, fruit juices without pulp, carbonated beverages, clear tea, and black coffee) or 6 hours after a light meal (without fried or fatty foods or meat). For patients presenting without the recommended fasting period, the target level of sedation should be modified if possible (less sedation administered), the procedure delayed, or tracheal intubation considered.

## Monitoring

During sedation, the patient's ventilation should be monitored by observation or auscultation. Based on our clinical experience, capnography is recommended because it may decrease the risk of adverse outcome, especially with deep sedation, if the patient is physically separated from the caregiver or when ventilation cannot be directly visualized. Oxygenation should also be monitored via pulse oximetry. The early detection of hypoxemia may reduce the risk of stroke, cardiac arrest, and death. Supplemental oxygen should be considered for moderate sedation and should be administered for deep sedation, as well as for elderly patients and those with significant comorbidities. The patient's vital signs should at least be monitored at 5-minute intervals. Sedatives can blunt a patient's normal autonomic responses, leading to hypotension and bradycardia. Alternatively, inadequate sedation can lead to hypertension and tachycardia. Early detection and treatment of these changes may reduce the risk of adverse outcomes. Continuous electrocardiogram may reduce risks during deep sedation or during moderate sedation in patients with cardiac disease.

The assessment of a patient's response to verbal commands should be continuously evaluated during moderate sedation except in those patients who cannot respond appropriately (young children, mentally impaired, or uncooperative patients). During upper endoscopy, a verbal response is not possible and, thus, a squeezing of the hand to verbal or tactile stimulation may be elicited to ensure the patient can control his or her airway and take deep breaths if necessary (corresponding to a state of moderate sedation). A response limited to reflex withdrawal from pain represents a state of general anesthesia.

# Commonly Used Sedation Drugs and Pharmacology

Evidence is mixed, but topical anesthetics may be useful as an adjunct to improve patient tolerance of endoscopy. The choice of sedation will depend on the patient and procedure to be performed and should be dosed with careful titration due to wide variability in patient response, as well as to allow for the delayed onset of some medications.

## OPIOIDS

Opioids are useful in improving a patient's tolerance of endoscopy, but it is important to remember that opioids do not provide amnesia by themselves. The major side effect of opioid administration is respiratory depression, which is exacerbated by coadministration of other sedatives. Nausea and vomiting are common side effects.

### Meperidine

Meperidine is a commonly used mu antagonist, and it is important to note that normeperidine, a long-lived metabolite of meperidine, is pro-convulsant. Especially with accumulation in the setting of renal failure, it may precipitate seizures (often preceded by irritability and tremor). Naloxone will not treat these seizures and may exacerbate seizure activity. Meperidine should be avoided in patients taking monoamine oxidase inhibitors (MAOIs), due to the risk for a life-threatening drug interaction that can include hypertensive crisis, hyperpyrexia, and cardiovascular collapse. Meperidine's duration of action is 1 to 3 hours and may prolong recovery in comparison to agents with a shorter duration of action.

### Fentanyl

Fentanyl has a more rapid onset (2 to 3 minutes) and shorter duration of action (30 minutes) than meperidine. Fentanyl, and its derivatives, can cause centrally mediated chest-wall rigidity, which may make ventilation difficult. Fentanyl can cause bradycardia, and while blood pressure remains remarkably stable with fentanyl administered alone, significant cardiovascular depression can occur if given in combination with benzodiazepines.

## NALOXONE

Naloxone is an opioid antagonist that can be used to reverse ventilatory depression (as well as analgesia) from an opioid overdose; 40 mcg should be administered every 2 to 3 minutes until the desired effect is obtained. Due to naloxone's short half-life (30 to 40 minutes), repeat doses may be necessary after 20 to 30 minutes if used to reverse an opioid with a longer half-life. For this reason, patients receiving naloxone should be monitored for an extended period of time (up to 2 hours). In patients chronically dependent on opioids, naloxone can precipitate acute withdrawal. Abrupt reversal has been associated with sympathetic outflow and pulmonary edema; therefore, slow titration is recommended.

## MIDAZOLAM

Due to its more rapid onset of action and shorter duration of action, midazolam is the benzodiazepine of choice for endoscopic sedation. The onset of action is 1 to 2 minutes, and the duration of effect is 20 to 80 minutes. Doses should be titrated every 2 minutes until the desired level of sedation achieved. In older adults, or in those with hepatic or renal impairment, smaller doses are recommended. Midazolam is superior to diazepam for endoscopic sedation because it has been shown to result in a faster onset of sedation, improved patient tolerance and more amnesia, fewer adverse events, and a comparable recovery profile. Midazolam, in combination with an opioid, can result in significant respiratory depression and even apnea. This apnea can occur some time after the last dose of midazolam was administered. Some patients may experience a paradoxical reaction to midazolam, with disinhibition and aggression.

## FLUMAZENIL

Flumazenil is a competitive gamma-aminobutyric acid antagonist used to reverse the effects of benzodiazepines. It is more effective at reversing sedation and amnesia than respiratory depression. Just as with naloxone for opioids, the duration of action of flumazenil (1 hour) can be shorter than the duration of even midazolam. Thus, additional dosing of flumazenil may be required. Flumazenil should be given in 0.2 mg-doses every minute (up to 3 mg total) until the desired level of reversal is achieved. Administration of flumazenil can cause seizures in patients who rely on benzodiazepines for the control of seizures or who are physically dependent on benzodiazepines. Vomiting and dizziness are 2 of the more frequently reported adverse reactions.

Most nonanesthesiologists rely on a combination of a benzodiazepine and an opioid. These regimens for moderate sedation seem to be effective and safe. There is evidence that the combination of midazolam and fentanyl, as compared to midazolam and meperidine, is associated with equal effectiveness but significantly shorter recovery time as long as excessive amounts of midazolam are not used (4 mg). Propofol likely results in the quickest recovery times.

## PROPOFOL

Propofol is a short-acting IV hypnotic agent that can be used for sedation at low doses or to induce general anesthesia at higher doses. Because of its rapid onset (30 to 60 seconds) and quick recovery profile (duration of action 4 to 8 minutes), propofol is increasingly being used for procedural sedation. Propofol also does not induce nausea, unlike opioids and many other sedatives. Although a patient with egg or soy allergy may not necessarily be allergic to propofol, the manufacturer states these allergies as contraindications. Propofol should not be used in patients with disorders of lipid metabolism or mitochondrial disease. Because of the concern for microbial contamination and sepsis, strict aseptic technique should be observed, and open propofol vials should be discarded after 6 hours.

Propofol is a cardiac depressant and lowers systemic vascular resistance. It also causes respiratory depression. For these reasons, careful patient monitoring is required during its use, and those administering propofol should be properly trained. While propofol has been administered by endoscopists as well as dedicated nurses, the US Food and Drug Administration (FDA) product label states "propofol should be administered only by persons trained in the administration of general anesthesia."

While many providers use propofol as the sole agent for sedation, it does not provide analgesia, and a deep sedation may be required for a patient to tolerate endoscopy. A moderate sedation may be difficult to achieve with propofol alone, as without large amounts of propofol, the patient may have significant movement or coughing during manipulation of the endoscope.

A balanced anesthetic, combining propofol with small doses of opioid or a benzodiazepine, may be beneficial in reducing the amount of propofol needed and, thus, potential side effects. With care, it may therefore be possible to target a level of moderate sedation with analgesia and amnesia provided by the other agents.

## FOSPROPOFOL

Fospropofol, a water-soluble prodrug of propofol, is a new agent that is converted into propofol by the liver. After a bolus of propofol is given, a lower peak level is obtained, and there is a longer duration of action. Due to its formulation, fospropofol may cause less pain on injection and a reduced chance of bacteremia. With an onset of action of at least 4 minutes, fospropofol takes significantly longer to take effect than propofol. Similar to propofol, fospropofol can cause respiratory depression, hypoxemia, and hypotension. Due to its delayed onset of action and prolonged effect, extra care is warranted with the administration of fospropofol.

## ADJUNCTIVE AGENTS

Other agents, such as droperidol, diphenhydramine, and promethazine are sometimes used as adjunctive agents.

### Droperidol

Droperidol is an antiemetic and central nervous system depressant. Its onset is 3 to 10 minutes, and duration of action is 2 to 4 hours. The usual dose for sedation is higher than that typically used for antiemetic effect. The main side effects include hypotension, prolonged $QT_C$ interval, and extrapyramidal reactions. In 2001, the FDA issued a black box warning for droperidol due to the risk for serious pro-arrhythmic effects and even death. The FDA also removed the use of droperidol as an adjunct for sedation from its list of indications. For these reasons, along with its prolonged duration of effect, droperidol is not recommended for routine use.

### Diphenhydramine

Diphenhydramine is an antihistamine that can be given intravenously as an adjunct for sedation. Its onset of action is on the order of 2 to 3 minutes, but peak effect may take 60 to 90 minutes. The duration of action is quite prolonged at 4 to 6 hours. It does not cause ventilatory depression, but side effects include hypotension, dizziness, blurry vision, dry mouth, epigastric pain, and urinary retention.

### Promethazine

Promethazine is a phenothiazine that, in addition to its antiemetic effect, can be used for sedation as an adjunct. It should be diluted and given slowly, with a careful eye on the injection site due to the risk of hypotension and severe tissue toxicity with extravasation. The onset of action is 5 minutes, and similar to the other described adjuncts, the duration of action is prolonged at 4 to 6 hours. Other side effects include respiratory depression, neuroleptic malignant syndrome, and extrapyramidal symptoms.

Based on the limited data available, these adjunctive agents may provide a small benefit for difficult sedations but, due to their significant side effects and prolonged duration of action, they likely should not be used routinely as the initial medications for standard endoscopies.

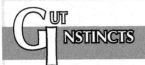

SEDATION

1. Sedation-related complications account for a large percentage of serious adverse events associated with endoscopy.

2. Most patients can successfully undergo endoscopic procedures under moderate sedation, but deep sedation or general anesthesia administered by an anesthesiologist may be preferable for certain patients or procedures.

3. Frequent assessment of vital signs and the depth of sedation via verbal or tactile stimulation are critical, and capnography is highly recommended.

4. Regimens combining a benzodiazepine and an opioid have proven to be safe and effective with the combination of midazolam and fentanyl showing the best recovery profile.

5. Propofol alone, or in combination with other agents, may provide superior patient and endoscopist satisfaction, as well as the quickest recovery and discharge times.

## Key References

1. Cohen LB, DeLegge MH, Aisenberg J, et al. AGA Institute review of endoscopic sedation. *Gastroenterology*. 2007;133(2):675-701.

2. American Society of Anesthesiologists Task Force on Sedation and Analgesia by Non-Anesthesiologists. Practice guidelines for sedation and analgesia by non-anesthesiologists. *Anesthesiology*. 2002;96(4):1004-1017.

3. McQuaid KR, Laine L. A systematic review and meta-analysis of randomized, controlled trials of moderate sedation for routine endoscopic procedures. *Gastrointestinal Endoscopy*. 2008;67(6):910-923.

CHAPTER **44**

# ANTICOAGULATION AND ANTIBIOTICS IN ENDOSCOPY

Kevin A. Ghassemi, MD

Endoscopic procedures carry small, but not insignificant, risks of bleeding and infection. Bleeding potential is increased in patients taking antithrombotic agents for various conditions. The endoscopist must decide whether to continue such medications periprocedurally in the face of a greater bleeding potential or to discontinue them and risk a thrombotic event. Infections can arise from bacteremia that results from mucosal trauma during endoscopy, or they can occur when normally sterile spaces are contaminated during endoscopic instrumentation. Bacteremia can occur in up to 50% of cases, depending on the procedure. In comparison, bacterial translocation from daily activities, such as brushing/flossing teeth and chewing food, can be more than 50%, yet antibiotics are not routinely given in these situations. Various factors must be considered to effectively perform endoscopic procedures and minimize the risks of bleeding, thrombosis, and infection.

## Anticoagulation

When deciding how to best take care of a patient on an antithrombotic agent who needs an endoscopic procedure, 4 simple questions need to be answered: (1) what is the patient taking? (2) why is the patient taking it? (3) when does the procedure need to be done? (4) how much bleeding risk is associated with the planned procedure?

Esrailian E. *Gut Instincts: A Clinician's Handbook of Digestive and Liver Diseases* (pp 313-318).
© 2012 Taylor & Francis Group

## WHAT? ANTITHROMBOTIC AGENTS

There are 2 major types of antithrombotic medications: antiplatelet agents that have duration of action of 5 to 10 days (aspirin/nonsteroidal anti-inflammatory drugs [NSAIDs]/clopidogrel) and anticoagulants (warfarin). There are no quick reversal agents for antiplatelet medications other than to transfuse platelets. Warfarin lasts approximately 3 to 5 days and can be reversed with either vitamin K or transfusion of fresh frozen plasma.

## WHY? INDICATION FOR ANTITHROMBOTIC AGENT

The majority of patients take antithrombotic agents for chronic indications. Patients with low-risk conditions (deep venous thrombosis, mechanical aortic valve, bioprosthetic valve, and uncomplicated/paroxysmal nonvalvular atrial fibrillation) have a thromboembolic event (TE) risk of about 1% if anticoagulation is held for 4 to 7 days. The risk is higher in patients on antithrombotic medications for the following conditions:

- Acute coronary syndrome
- Recent coronary stent placement (less than 1 year)
- Percutaneous coronary intervention after a myocardial infarction
- Mechanical mitral valve
- Mechanical valve in any position and a prior TE
- Complicated atrial fibrillation (age >75, diabetes, hypertension, prior TE, valvular heart disease, prosthetic valve, active congestive heart failure, or left ventricular ejection fraction <35%).

## WHEN? PROCEDURE URGENCY

The degree of urgency to perform an endoscopic procedure will help dictate whether the effect of the antithrombotic agent needs to be reversed. The main reasons for a procedure to be performed urgently are significant acute bleeding, acute cholangitis, and foreign-body retrieval. Other endoscopic procedures typically are performed as elective cases.

## HOW? PROCEDURE BLEEDING RISK

With the exception of mucosal biopsy, any procedure that involves cutting, hemostasis, or dilation will have a high bleeding risk. This includes polypectomy, sphincterotomy, treatment of gastrointestinal (GI) bleeding, dilation, percutaneous endoscopic gastrostomy (PEG) placement, and endoscopic ultrasound (EUS) with fine-needle aspiration (FNA).

Diagnostic procedures generally are considered low-risk procedures and include esophagogastroduodenoscopy/colonoscopy/enteroscopy with mucosal biopsy, endoscopic retrograde cholangiopancreatography (ERCP) without sphincterotomy, EUS without FNA, and capsule endoscopy. Additionally, enteral stent placement is also a low-risk procedure if it is not performed along with dilation.

## Antithrombotic Management Recommendations

- For low-risk procedures, regardless of urgency, continue the antithrombotic agent
- For high-risk procedures and low TE risk, regardless of urgency:
  - Consider continuing aspirin/NSAIDs
  - Hold clopidogrel for 7 to 10 days, or as long as possible if urgent
- For high-risk procedures in patients on clopidogrel:
  - Consider postponing elective procedures until the TE risk is low
  - Hold clopidogrel for urgent procedures
- Discontinue warfarin for all high-risk procedures, and consider bridging therapy with unfractionated heparin (UFH) or low molecular weight heparin (LMWH)
- The decision of when to restart antithrombotic medications should be individualized:
  - For high TE risk, UFH or LMWH may be used in the immediate post-procedure period
  - For low TE risk, warfarin usually can be resumed the same evening that the procedure was performed

## Antibiotics

Infections can occur when mucosal disruption occurs or when sterile spaces are contaminated. Important factors to consider include the chance of an infection occurring, the potential clinical consequences if the infection occurs, and what type of antibiotic coverage would be appropriate. These issues are described below and are summarized in Table 44-1.

### ENDOSCOPIC RETROGRADE CHOLANGIOPANCREATOGRAPHY

The biliary tree is a sterile area. The contrast that is injected for cholangiography is not sterile, and this represents a potential source

| TABLE 44-1 | RECOMMENDATIONS FOR ANTIBIOTIC PROPHYLAXIS IN ENDOSCOPIC PROCEDURES | | |
|---|---|---|---|
| **Procedure** | **Condition** | **Prophylaxis?** | **Antibiotic** |
| Any prodecure | Any cardiac | No* | - |
| | Prosthetic device | No | - |
| | Cirrhosis + GI bleed | On admission, continue for 7 days | Ceftriaxone 1 g IV, norfloxacin 2nd line |
| ERCP | Complete biliary drainage | No | GN/enterococcal coverage |
| | Incomplete biliary drainage | Until drained | GN/enterococcal coverage |
| ERCP/EUS | Drainage of sterile pancreatic fluid collection | 3 days | Fluoroquinolone |
| EUS-FNA | UGI solid lesion | No | - |
| | LGI solid lesion | 3 days | Fluoroquinolone |
| | Cystic lesion | 3-5 days | Fluoroquinolone |
| PEG | - | 30 minutes before | IV 1st-gen cephalosporin, vancomycin if MRSA |

*In high-risk cardiac conditions, prophylaxis with enterococcal coverage should be used.

GN indicates gram negative; UGI, upper gastrointestinal; LGI, lower gastrointestinal; PEG, percutaneous endoscopic gastrostomy

of infection. Acute cholangitis can be life threatening if not treated urgently. However, as long as the contrast is able to drain completely, the risk of cholangitis and sepsis is very low. Incomplete drainage is the most predictive factor of infectious complications. Therefore, in noncholangitis cases when complete biliary drainage is anticipated (eg, choledocholithiasis), prophylactic antibiotics are not necessary. When complete drainage is less likely, such as primary sclerosing cholangitis (PSC) or a malignant hilar stricture, antibiotic prophylaxis should be administered and continued until complete drainage can be achieved. The biliary tree typically is infected by enteric gram-negative (GN) bacteria and enterococci, so antibiotics should cover these organisms.

## ENDOSCOPIC ULTRASOUND-GUIDED FINE-NEEDLE ASPIRATION

The risk of infection with EUS-FNA depends on the reason for the FNA. When it is performed on solid lesions in the upper GI tract, the infection rate is very low, and antibiotic prophylaxis is not warranted. The data to determine the risk of infection from FNA of lower GI tract solid lesions thus far are insufficient; therefore, antibiotic prophylaxis with a fluoroquinolone for 3 days may be considered. For cystic lesions along the GI tract, the infection rate can be approximately 10%. Studies have shown that fluoroquinolones significantly reduced the rate of infection, and they are recommended for 3 to 5 days when FNA is performed on cystic lesions.

## PERCUTANEOUS ENDOSCOPIC GASTROSTOMY

There is a high incidence of peristomal infections when prophylactic antibiotics are not used for percutaneous feeding tube placement. Antibiotics that cover skin flora (eg, first-generation cephalosporins) have been shown to significantly reduce the infection rate. With the increase in antibiotic resistance, patients with documented methicillin-resistant *Staphylococcus aureus* infection/colonization should receive vancomycin instead. Intravenous antibiotics should be administered 30 minutes before PEG-tube placement.

# Cardiac Conditions

Only the highest-risk cardiac conditions, defined by the American Heart Association, should be considered for antibiotic prophylaxis. These conditions include prior infective endocarditis, prosthetic valve, congenital heart disease, and heart transplant with valvulopathy. If patients have any of these conditions in the setting of a suspected enterococcal GI tract infection, enterococcal coverage should be considered.

# Cirrhotic Patients With Gastrointestinal Bleeding

The risk of bacteremia is increased in patients with cirrhosis and GI bleeding because of altered intestinal permeability and increased bacterial translocation across the GI tract. Aerobic GN bacteria are the usual isolated organism. Therefore, all cirrhotic patients with GI bleeding, regardless of procedure planned, should receive an intravenous third-generation cephalosporin upon presentation.

## Prosthetic Devices

There are very few reports of infections affecting these devices as a result of endoscopic procedures. Antibiotic prophylaxis is not recommended in these cases.

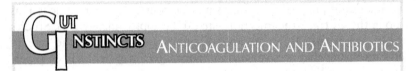

1. Antithrombotic agents can be continued in the setting of endoscopic procedures with low bleeding risks.
2. For high-risk procedures, aspirin generally can be continued, but clopidogrel should be discontinued if possible.
3. Patients taking warfarin who need to undergo a high-risk procedure should stop the warfarin beforehand. Bridging therapy should be used if there is a high risk of a thromboembolic event with stopping anticoagulation.
4. Most cases of endoscopic instrumentation of a sterile space will require antibiotic prophylaxis with the exception of complete biliary drainage during endoscopic retrograde cholangiopancreatography.
5. Cirrhotic patients with gastrointestinal bleeding need antibiotic prophylaxis regardless of the endoscopic procedure planned.

## Key References

1. ASGE Standards of Practice Committee. Management of antithrombotic agents for endoscopic procedures. *Gastrointest Endosc.* 2009;70(6): 1060-1070.
2. ASGE Standards of Practice Committee. Antibiotic prophylaxis for GI endoscopy. *Gastrointest Endosc.* 2008;67(6):791-798.

# CHAPTER 45

# BOWEL PREPARATIONS
# FOR COLONOSCOPY

Wendy Ho, MD, MPH

Colonoscopy is the most common procedure used to evaluate the colon, and preparation quality is a critical component of this procedure. For colonoscopy to be successful, the colon must be cleansed of all stool so the mucosa can be adequately examined. If the colon is not appropriately cleansed, colonoscopy is often more difficult and requires a longer procedure time. In some cases, the bowel preparation and colonoscopy even need to be repeated, effectively doubling the expense and inconvenience to patients. Finally, poor colon preparation can result in missed lesions and increased complication rates. There are many different colon preparation techniques that have been developed. The ideal colon preparation would be easily accessible, easy to use, effective, and safe. Table 45-1 provides a summary of advantages and disadvantages of common bowel preparations.

## Polyethylene Glycol (PEG: Colyte and GoLYTELY)

Polyethylene glycol (Colyte, Kaiser Permanente, Oakland, CA and GoLYTELY, Braintree Labs, Braintree, MA) is a nonabsorbable electrolyte lavage solution that passes through the bowel without net absorption or secretion. It is effective and safe. It consists of 4 L of PEG solution that can be consumed either the night prior to the procedure or as part of a divided dose administration with patients drinking 2 to

Esrailian E. *Gut Instincts: A Clinician's Handbook of Digestive and Liver Diseases* (pp 319-324).
© 2012 Taylor & Francis Group

| TABLE 45-1 | SUMMARY OF ADVANTAGES AND DISADVANTAGES OF COMMON BOWEL PREPARATIONS | |
|---|---|---|
| **Name** | **Advantages** | **Disadvantages** |
| Polyethylene glycol (polyethylene glycol [PEG], Colyte, Kaiser Permanente, Oakland, CA; GoLYTELY, Braintree Labs, Braintree, MA) | Safe | Large volume, poor taste |
| Sulfate-free PEG (NuLYTELY, Braintree Labs, Braintree, MA; TriLyte, Schwarz Pharma for Alaven Pharmaceutical, LLC, Marietta, GA) | Safe, better taste | Large volume |
| Low-volume PEG and bisacodyl (HalfLYTELY, Braintree Labs, Braintree, MA) | Safe, lower volume | 2 L solution still a sizeable volume to drink |
| Low-volume sulfate solution (SUPREP, Braintree Labs, Braintree, MA) | Lower volume | Risk of electrolyte fluctuation and use caution in renal dysfunction |
| Ascorbic acid lavage (MoviPrep, Salix Pharmaceuticals, Inc, Morrisville, NC) | Safe, better taste | Use with caution in patients with G6PD deficiency |
| Hyperosmolar laxatives | None | Bacterial fermentation of carbohydrates carries risk of explosion during electrocautery |
| Sodium phosphate • Liquid form • Visicol tablets (Salix Pharmaceuticals, Inc, Morrisville, NC) • OsmoPrep tablets (Salix Pharmaceuticals, Inc, Morrisville, NC) | Small volume of oral preparation ingestion | Requires high concomitant liquid ingestion. Caution in cardiac/liver/renal dysfunction; elderly/dehydrated, those taking angiotensin-converting enzyme inhibitors or angiotensin receptor blockers |
| Magnesium citrate as adjunct to PEG | Lower volume of PEG required | Caution in renal dysfunction |
| Rectal pulsed irritation | Low volume of prep ingestion | Not routinely offered due to cost/requirement for skilled nursing |

3 L of PEG the night before colonoscopy and another 1 to 2 L the morning of colonoscopy. The divided dose administration increases patient tolerance and the quality of bowel preparation. Split dosing may be difficult to do for morning procedures, but it should be considered for all afternoon procedures or for patients with a history of constipation. The disadvantages of PEG include its salty taste and large volume, which can cause bloating and fullness, to the point that some patients do not complete the preparation.

## Sulfate-Free PEG (NuLYTELY and TriLyte)

Sulfate-free PEG preparations (NuLYTELY, Braintree Labs, Braintree, MA and TriLyte, Schwarz Pharma for Alaven Pharmaceutical, LLC, Marietta, GA) are similar to PEG with improved taste due to the elimination of sodium sulfate, decreased potassium, and increased chloride. The taste might be more acceptable to patients. These are similar to PEG in all other respects (4 L volume and similar safety and effectiveness).

## Low-Volume PEG and Bisacodyl (HalfLYTELY)

Low-volume PEG and bisacodyl preparation (HalfLYTELY, Braintree Labs, Braintree, MA) consists of 2 L PEG taken with bisacodyl tablets. Patients take bisacodyl 20 mg, wait for either the first bowel movement or 6 hours, and then take the 2 L of PEG. This gives similar colon preparation results as compared to 4 L PEG, but with improved patient tolerance.

## Low-Volume Sulfate Preparation

Low-volume sulfate preparation (SUPREP, Braintree Labs, Braintree, MA) is composed of a sodium, potassium, and magnesium sulfate solution given as a split-dose regimen. The first 6-ounce bottle is taken the night before the colonoscopy, and the second 6-ounce bottle is taken the following morning.

## Ascorbic Acid Lavage (MoviPrep)

Ascorbic acid lavage (MoviPrep, Salix Pharmaceuticals, Inc, Morrisville, NC) makes the bowel preparation more palatable and also acts as a cathartic agent. This is a 3-L bowel preparation with similar efficacy to a 4-L PEG solution. It should be used with caution in patients with glucose-6-phosphate dehydrogenase (G6PD) deficiency because high doses of ascorbic acid can induce hemolysis.

# Hyperosmolar Laxatives

Mannitol, sorbitol, and lactulose are nonabsorbable carbohydrates that are hyperosmolar laxatives. These are not often used for colon preparation due to bacterial fermentation into hydrogen and methane gas, which can cause intracolonic explosion during electrocautery.

# Sodium Phosphate

Sodium phosphate contains phosphate ions, which are hyperosmotic and cause water to be drawn into and retained in the gut lumen. This action stimulates stretch receptors and induces peristalsis. The liquid form must be diluted prior to ingestion and must be accompanied by oral fluid ingestion to prevent dehydration. It is taken in 2 doses of 30 to 45 mL, 10 to 12 hours apart. Each dose is taken with at least 8 ounces of liquid followed by a minimum of at least 16 ounces of additional liquid. This preparation can cause mucosal lesions that are similar to those seen in inflammatory bowel disease, nonsteroidal anti-inflammatory drug use, or other drug-induced lesions, and should be avoided in diagnostic colonoscopy in which inflammatory bowel disease or microscopic colitis is suspected. In addition, this bowel preparation can cause significant fluid and electrolyte changes and is, therefore, contraindicated in patients with heart failure, liver dysfunction, bowel obstruction, small intestine disorders, poor gut motility, renal dysfunction, dehydration, hypercalcemia, those taking angiotensin-converting enzyme inhibitors and angiotensin receptor blockers (can cause nephrocalcinosis), and elderly patients. Due to reports of acute phosphate nephropathy, the US Food and Drug Administration (FDA) has taken this product, as used for bowel preparation, off of the market. In addition, Visicol and OsmoPrep (both by Salix Pharmaceuticals, Inc, Morrisville, NC and both described below), as well as oral sodium phosphate, which is available without a prescription as a laxative, now carry an FDA black box warning.

The tablet form of sodium phosphate contains about the same amount of active ingredient as the standard liquid sodium phosphate regimen. These agents have a similar efficacy to PEG solutions and have fewer side effects. However, they have the same risks as liquid sodium phosphate preparations and, thus, must be used with caution.

### VISICOL

Visicol tablets (20 tablets taken both the evening before and the morning of the procedure) contain microcrystalline cellulose as a tablet binder. This binder is insoluble and can deposit in the colon, obscuring the colonic mucosa visibility.

## OSMOPREP

OsmoPrep tablets (20 tablets the evening before the procedure and 12 tablets the morning of the procedure) are a residue-free formulation of sodium phosphate and, thus, do not have the problem of poor mucosal visibility.

# Magnesium Citrate

Magnesium citrate is a saline laxative that relies on the hyperosmotic effect of poorly absorbed magnesium cations. It also causes cholecystokinin release, which increases small bowel, and possibly colonic, motility. Magnesium citrate 300 mL is sometimes used as an adjunct to PEG to decrease the volume of PEG required (2 L). It should be used with caution in patients with renal insufficiency.

# Rectal Pulsed Irritation

This method of colonic preparation is done with oral ingestion of 300 mL magnesium citrate the day prior to colonoscopy and rectal pulsed irrigation immediately before colonoscopy. The rectal irrigation consists of a 30-minute infusion of short pulses of tap water through a rectal tube. It is comparable to PEG with regard to colon cleansing. However, this modality is not offered routinely because it is time consuming, requires skilled nursing staff and special equipment, and is more expensive than a standard preparation.

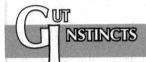

**BOWEL PREPARATIONS**

1. Poor colon preparation can result in missed lesions and increased complication rates.
2. Polyethylene glycol-based bowel preparation solutions are an effective and safe method for colon cleansing.
3. Divided-dosing polyethylene glycol gives better colon preparation and is better tolerated by patients. This should particularly be considered for patients having afternoon procedures.
4. Sodium phosphate-based bowel preparations should be used with caution in patients with comorbidities or when diagnostic colonoscopy is being done for suspected inflammatory bowel disease.
5. Consider tailoring the bowel preparation in patients with baseline constipation to avoid a suboptimal result.

## Key References

1. Hawes RH, Lowry A, Deziel D. A consensus document on bowel preparation before colonoscopy: prepared by a task force from the ASCRS, ASGE, and SAGES. *Gastrointest Endosc.* 2006;63(7):894-909.
2. Aon E, Abdul-Baki H, Azar C, et al. A randomized single-blind trial of split-dose PEG-electrolyte solution without dietary restriction compared with whole dose PEG-electrolyte solution with dietary restriction for colonoscopy preparation. *Gastrointest Endosc.* 2005;62(2):213-218.

# FINANCIAL DISCLOSURES

*Gillian M. Barlow, PhD* has no financial or proprietary interest in the materials presented herein.

*Simon W. Beaven, MD, PhD* has no financial or proprietary interest in the materials presented herein.

*Yasser M. Bhat, MD* has no financial or proprietary interest in the materials presented herein.

*Lin Chang, MD* received grant support from Takeda, and is a consultant for Ironwood, Takeda, Forest, and Albireo.

*William D. Chey, MD, AGAF, FACG, FACP* is a consultant for AstraZeneca and Takeda.

*Daniel D. Cho, MD* has no financial or proprietary interest in the materials presented herein.

*Jeffrey L. Conklin, MD, FACG* is a consultant for Given Imaging.

*Lynn Shapiro Connolly, MD* has no financial or proprietary interest in the materials presented herein.

*Stanley Dea, MD* has no financial or proprietary interest in the materials presented herein.

*John A. Donovan, MD* has no financial or proprietary interest in the materials presented herein.

*Marla Dubinsky, MD* received research support from Centocor Ortho Biotech and UCB. She is a consultant for Prometheus, Abbott, UCB, and Shire.

*John P. Duffy, MD* has no financial or proprietary interest in the materials presented herein.

*Francisco Antonio Durazo, MD, FACP* has no financial or proprietary interest in the materials presented herein.

*Erik P. Dutson, MD, FACS* has no financial or proprietary interest in the materials presented herein.

*Eric Esrailian, MD, MPH* has no financial or proprietary interest in the materials presented herein.

*James Farrell, MD* has no financial or proprietary interest in the materials presented herein.

*Terri Getzug, MD* has no financial or proprietary interest in the materials presented herein.

*Kevin A. Ghassemi, MD* has no financial or proprietary interest in the materials presented herein.

*Gary Gitnick, MD, FACG* has no financial or proprietary interest in the materials presented herein.

*Steven-Huy Han, MD, AGAF* is a consultant and on the speaker's bureau for Bristol-Myers Squibb and Gilead.

*O. Joe Hines, MD* has no financial or proprietary interest in the materials presented herein.

*Wendy Ho, MD, MPH* has no financial or proprietary interest in the materials presented herein.

*Ke-Qin Hu, MD* received grants from Bayer HealthCare, Bristol-Myers Squibb, Gilead Scientific, Novartis, Onyx, Genentech, Merck, and Vertex. Dr. Hu is also a member of the speaker bureau of Bristol-Myers Squibb, Bayer HealthCare, Genentech, Gilead Scientific, Onyx, Merck, and Vertex.

*Dennis M. Jensen, MD* received research grants from Olympus, Pentax, and Boston Scientific. Dr. Jensen is a consultant and on the speaker's bureau for US Endoscopy and Boston Scientific.

*Rome Jutabha, MD* has no financial or proprietary interest in the materials presented herein.

*Fasiha Kanwal, MS, MSHS* has no financial or proprietary interest in the materials presented herein.

*Theodoros Kelesidis, MD* has no financial or proprietary interest in the materials presented herein.

*Saro Khemichian, MD* has no financial or proprietary interest in the materials presented herein.

*Vandana Khungar, MD, MSc* has no financial or proprietary interest in the materials presented herein.

*Kunut Kijsirichareanchai, MD* has no financial or proprietary interest in the materials presented herein.

*Thomas O. G. Kovacs, MD* has no financial or proprietary interest in the materials presented herein.

*Amy Lightner, MD* has no financial or proprietary interest in the materials presented herein.

*Emeran A. Mayer, MD* has no financial or proprietary interest in the materials presented herein.

*Gil Y. Melmed, MD, MS* is a consultant for Centocor, Amgen, and Celgene, and is on the speaker's bureau for Prometheus Labs.

*Michel H. Mendler, MD, MS* has no financial or proprietary interest in the materials presented herein.

*Lilah F. Morris, MD* has no financial or proprietary interest in the materials presented herein.

*Udayakumar Navaneethan, MD* has no financial or proprietary interest in the materials presented herein.

*Vivian Ng, MD* has no financial or proprietary interest in the materials presented herein.

*Mark Ovsiowitz, MD* has no financial or proprietary interest in the materials presented herein.

*David A. Pegues, MD* has no financial or proprietary interest in the materials presented herein.

*Mark Pimentel, MD, FRCP(C)* received grants from Salix and the Beatrice and Samuel A. Seaver Foundation, and is a consultant for Salix. Dr. Pimentel works at Cedars-Sinai Medical Center which has a licensing agreement with Salix.

*Charalabos Pothoulakis, MD* is a consultant for Optimer, Biocodex, and Robert Michael Educational Institute, LLC.

*Bennett E. Roth, MD* has no financial or proprietary interest in the materials presented herein.

*Bruce A. Runyon, MD* is a consultant for Ikaria and NovaShunt.

*Sammy Saab, MD, MPH, AGAF* has no financial or proprietary interest in the materials presented herein.

*Richard J. Saad, MD, MS* has no financial or proprietary interest in the materials presented herein.

*Jonathan Sack, MD* has no financial or proprietary interest in the materials presented herein.

*Saeed Sadeghi, MD* is on the speaker's bureau for Genentech.

*Bo Shen, MD, FACG* has no financial or proprietary interest in the materials presented herein.

*Inder M. Singh, MD* has no financial or proprietary interest in the materials presented herein.

*Tram T. Tran, MD* has no financial or proprietary interest in the materials presented herein.

*Leo Treyzon, MD, MS* has no financial or proprietary interest in the materials presented herein.

*Zev A. Wainberg, MD, MSc* has no financial or proprietary interest in the materials presented herein.

*Samuel H. Wald, MD* has no financial or proprietary interest in the materials presented herein.

*Wilfred M. Weinstein, MD* has no financial or proprietary interest in the materials presented herein.

*Jeremy M. Wong, MD* has no financial or proprietary interest in the materials presented herein.

*James Yoo, MD, FACS, FASCRS* has no financial or proprietary interest in the materials presented herein.

*David Da Zheng, BS* has no financial or proprietary interest in the materials presented herein.

# INDEX

Printed in the United States
by Baker & Taylor Publisher Services